STRENGTH TRAINING
for the Martial Arts

TONY GUMMERSON

A & C Black · London

First published 1990 by
A & C Black (Publishers) Ltd
35 Bedford Row, London WC1R 4JH

© 1990 Tony Gummerson

ISBN 0 7136 3263 1

A CIP catalogue record for this book is
available from the British Library.

Typeset by Latimer Trend & Company
Ltd, Plymouth
Printed and bound in Great Britain by
BPCC Hazell Books, Aylesbury, Bucks

CONTENTS

ACKNOWLEDGEMENTS

The production of this book was made possible by the help and encouragement of many martial artists. In particular I would like to thank:

Steve Hateley of the British Thai Boxing Council, who provided considerable technical input and made available the use of his club and facilities at Extremeties, Middleton, Manchester

David Mitchell, who was instrumental in setting up the Martial Arts Commission Coach Education Programme and creating an interest in applying sports science to the martial arts

Peter and *Gary* for their patience in demonstrating the various excercises.

I would also like to thank Martin Sellars for the photographs.

Note

Throughout the book students and coaches are, in the main, referred to individually as 'he'. This should, of course, be taken to mean 'he or she' where appropriate.

INTRODUCTION

Throughout humanity's evolution men and women have constantly tested their intellect and physical prowess against both the environment and other individuals. Out of this 'live-or-die' situation emerged two distinct areas for the application of their talents. Firstly, they had the important task of surviving the ravages of the elements and, secondly, they had to defend themselves from or attack others.

In the history and mythology of all races there have been heroes whose physical prowess and expertise in battle have become legendary. However, as human beings have evolved, civilisation and mechanisation have largely taken away the demand for personal fighting skills. Paradoxically, while the need for hand-to-hand combat has declined, the martial arts, as a sporting and recreational activity, have flourished. They have offered the opportunity for individuals to emulate the heroes of old in the development of the highest levels of technical mastery of the fighting arts.

The martial arts have progressed in such a way that they now give students the chance to learn traditional techniques, and to submit themselves to rigorous physical and mental training in a safe environment. Through carefully designed syllabuses, grading systems and competitions students can identify a particular element of the martial arts which appeals specifically to them. From tai chi to full-contact karate there will be one martial art or style which is appropriate to their needs.

Martial arts, particularly over the past twenty years, have attracted an ever-increasing number of followers. Many have been drawn by their visions of Bruce Lee and other film and video stars, but perhaps more surprisingly many have been attracted by the mystique surrounding the arts. In today's hedonistic way of life students have sought a kind of escape, be it physical, religious or philosophical. Whatever an individual's reason for becoming a martial arts student, each person will undoubtedly achieve personal development through training.

The present standards of technical excellence in the martial arts are based on the evolution of traditional techniques. However, many of the training methods and practices advocated in the past would be unacceptable today. It seems appropriate, therefore, that as many of the arts are reassessing their own philosophies and values, they should also be reappraising their training methods. In the past twenty or so years increasing interest has been shown in the application of both science and medicine to sport. Out of this trend have emerged two disciplines: 'sports sciences' and 'sports medicine'. So, although the current state of the martial arts is firmly rooted in history, their continued development and credibility depend upon a willingness to adopt new practices and methods.

Sports scientists identify very specific areas which require particular attention, but the committed coach has to apply theories to the 'real' world. In terms of their practical implication, sports medicine and science can be encapsulated in the notion of the 'S' factors:

- speed
- strength
- stamina
- suppleness
- skill
- 'p'sychology

For speed, muscles have to contract quickly to move a limb or the whole body at the fastest possible rate. For endurance, muscles have to be able to work over a long period of time, even when fatigue starts to develop. Suppleness depends upon muscles moving a limb through a set range of movement required by a particular action. Skilful performance results from muscles producing force in a precise way that is appropriate to the action. This might range from the generation of power in the shortest possible time, for example in breaking techniques, to the sustained delicate movements of tai chi.

For the correct application of all 'S' factors, 'p'sychology is essential. The individual must have the appropriate level of commitment, dedication and enthusiasm for his own particular style. The coach must ensure that for each student the best possible teaching and learning situation is created.

The contribution which the 'S' factors make to the overall excellence of performance will be peculiar to each art or style. It therefore must fall to the coach to identify how much emphasis on the separate elements there should be in training. He must choose those elements that are appropriate not only for the style being taught, but also for the individual needs of his students.

Each of the 'S' factors should really be included in any training session, irrespective of their degree of importance. This is the coach's dilemma! However, one of the more basic elements is 'strength', since all activity in one's daily life or sport ultimately depends on the contraction of muscles for its source of power.

When designing training programmes the coach must consider carefully both the technical requirements of his style and the level of strength needed for excellence of performance. He should ask himself:

- what type of strength do particular techniques require?
- which exercises will develop that strength?

The following chapters look at the types of strength and their application to martial arts. The development of precise aspects of strength acquisition will be discussed. The very nature of strength is identified so that the theory behind a training programme can be appreciated.

MUSCLE TISSUE

All of the physical controls which maintain the function of internal organs and the general well-being of the individual depend upon muscles working effectively. Muscle activity may involve: movement of the whole body or just part of it; the digestion of food; the beating of the heart and the direction of blood to specific parts of the body; and many other processes.

In the human body there are basically three types of muscle tissue which are responsible for these functions. They are as follows.

Smooth muscle

This is found mostly in the internal organs and surrounding blood vessels. Its main purpose is to provide the power for the digestive process and to control the volume of blood flowing into specific areas of the body. Generally speaking, it plays a vital role in maintaining the body in a healthy state. Since many of its functions are of a routine nature, they are not controlled in a conscious manner but are governed by that part of the brain which operates such functions in an 'automatic' fashion.

Cardiac muscle

As its name implies, this is only found in the heart. The heart is a muscular pump which supplies blood at a rate which will provide the necessary oxygen and nutrients for growth and for the demands of physical activity. It is a very versatile organ in that it can increase or decrease its work rate according to the demands being placed upon the body. It also has a unique feature: unlike other muscular tissue which has to be stimulated by the nervous system to contract, cardiac muscle possesses 'autorhythmicity', i.e. the ability to function independently of external stimulation. The control of heart rate is too important to leave to the conscious part of the brain since it might forget to 'tell' the heart to beat! So, the very delicate controlling mechanisms which allow the heart to function in a manner appropriate to the varying workloads put on it are looked after mainly by the subconscious part of the brain.

Skeletal muscle

These muscles bring about movement in 'co-operation' with the skeletal system. By and large they are under direct conscious control and, certainly in the field of physical activity, their function is critical. It is skeletal muscle which is responsible for the production of movement in general and skilful performance in particular.

Although the function of smooth and cardiac muscle is essential for any physical activity, in the development of strength for the refinement of technique skeletal muscle plays the main role. All of the exercises and training programmes described in this book are therefore aimed specifically at skeletal muscle.

HOW MUSCLES WORK

Muscles usually generate movement or force by contracting. This action normally brings about a pulling on that part of the skeleton to which the muscle is attached, and in the process movement occurs.

Muscles need a very efficient blood transport system which can provide the required oxygen and nutrients to produce the energy for physical activity. At the same time they must be able to remove carbon dioxide and other waste products. In order to do this, blood supplied from the heart by arteries is dispersed through the muscle tissue by much smaller vessels or capillaries. The blood then picks up the carbon dioxide and waste products, and returns them to the veins where they are taken away for processing or elimination.

Having energy available to do useful work, however, is not enough: there has to be some kind of mechanism for regulating the contraction of the muscle. This is achieved by a series of 'motor nerves' which transmit instructions from the Central Nervous System (CNS), i.e. the brain and the spinal column. For the brain to co-ordinate movement it needs to have knowledge of the length of the muscle and the amount of force it is generating. Within the muscle and its tendon attachments to the bone there are special sensory organs which provide this necessary information.

THE STRUCTURE AND FUNCTION OF MUSCLES

Though the structure of a muscle may, on the face of it, seem very complex, it is, in fact, one of nature's attempts to resolve a difficult problem.

Apart from the skin, which is not actually attached to the muscle, the outermost structure responsible for its shape is the **epimysium**. This membrane merges at each end into the tendons which convert the force of muscular contraction into movement.

In a cross-section of muscle, many individual fibres are grouped in **bundles**, each of which is separated from the others by a structure known as the **septum**. The bundles, also known as **fasciculi**, have their own surrounding membrane called the **perimysium**. Each bundle may contain between 12–150 fibres, and has its own individual membrane known as the **endomysium**.

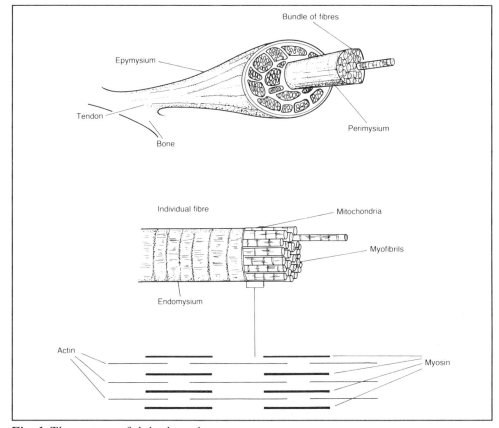

Fig. 1 *The structure of skeletal muscle*

Shortening a muscle

The need for this series of sheaths of tissue which surround the

- single fibre (**endomysium**)
- bundles of fibres (**perimysium**)
- whole muscle (**epimysium**)

might be better understood if it is realised that, by and large, fibres do not run the entire length of the **fasciculus**. The fasciluli do not necessarily run the length of the muscle either. There has to be some mechanism, therefore, which allows the contraction of individual fibres to have an effect on the muscle as a whole. The series of events can be broken down as follows.

1 The individual fibre contracts, causing the **endomysium** to shorten.
2 Since the endomysium connects fibres to each other in a **fasciculus**, when an individual fibre contracts the whole unit shortens (even though the other fibres may not be active). This series of events then causes the **perimysium** to shorten.
3 Because the separate bundles of fibres are enclosed by the **epimysium**, if any one of these contracts it brings about the shortening of the entire muscle.

Contraction processes

So far, the mechanics of how the muscle shortens have been described, but what are the actual processes by which it contracts?

Muscle fibres are relatively small structures. They are:

- 10–100 microns (1,000 microns = 1 mm) in diameter, and
- 1 mm to 30 cm in length.

The size, particularly the diameter, of each individual fibre is related to the type of force that it is required to produce. For example, the size of the single fibres in the quadriceps muscle of the upper thigh, which have to produce power, is larger than that of those responsible for movements of the eye. The dimensions of a large fibre are roughly similar to those of a single human hair, while the smaller ones are invisible to the naked eye.

Each muscle fibre is an individual cell surrounded by a membrane known as the **sarcolemma**. Running longitudinally along the length of the cell enclosed by the sarcolemma are thin column-like structures called **myofibrils**. These are made up of two types of protein, **actin** and **myosin**, which are responsible for the contraction of the cell and, because of the way in which they lay over each other, they produce dark and light bands. This striped appearance has given rise to skeletal muscles also being called **striated**.

These bands are at the very heart of the contractile mechanism. When a fibre is called upon to contract, the actin and myosin filaments slide over each other. Though neither actually changes in length, because of their movement in relation to one another, the overall effect is for the fibre to shorten.

Before a muscle can contract it requires a signal. The process by which signals are transmitted to muscles is usually referred to as **innervation**. **Motor nerves** pass on the necessary impulse from the Central Nervous System. The function of the muscle greatly affects how this mechanism works. For example, where a muscle is generally required to produce a large force, one motor nerve might be attached to several hundred individual muscle fibres. In such a case a single impulse would cause a hundred fibres to contract at the same time. However, where very delicate movements are required, such as with the eye, one motor nerve might be attached to only ten fibres.

With **skeletal** muscle tissue there is a further dimension to the way in which muscle fibres work. This is based on the fact that there are different types of fibre in any muscle, each having their own particular quality. These are as follows.

Slow twitch or red fibres

Such fibres are designed for endurance work, being able to sustain long periods of low intensity activity. They are particularly resistant to the build-up of waste products and associated fatigue. They are called 'slow twitch' because, as their name implies, they do not contract quickly. The 'red' description comes from the fact that they have a well-developed blood supply. This aspect is very important in that oxygen and nutrients are readily made available via the blood for long, sustained periods of work. Similarly, the waste products are removed as they are produced, thereby preventing any problems of fatigue.

Fast twitch or white fibres

These are designed for short periods of high intensity work. Although they will produce great amounts of force, they fatigue very quickly. 'Fast twitch' relates to the speed with which the fibres contract and the speed with which impulses via the motor nerves stimulate them into action. The 'white' description refers in part to the fact that there is a well-developed nervous system which aids the speed of contraction and innervation of the muscle. However, white fibres do not have a highly developed blood supply system and this reduces the rate of oxygen and nutrient transport. But, perhaps more importantly, it reduces the rate of waste product removal build-up, which is one of the major aspects of fatigue.

Intermediate fibres

The proportion of fast to slow twitch fibres in a muscle is governed at birth, though some people might dispute this! The characteristic would seem to identify those students who will have the potential for speed or endurance. Numerous studies have examined the fibre types of different sportsmen and

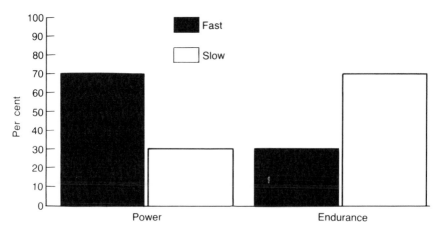

Fig. 2 *The distribution of muscle fibre types in athletes*

women, and have shown that individuals involved in power or speed events have a higher proportion of fast twitch fibres than those in endurance events who have more slow twitch fibres. More detailed results have been obtained in research undertaken to look at fibre distribution in athletes.

By considering the specific demands of individual martial arts with respect to leg, upper body or endurance strength, the requirements for excellence might be better understood. Does all this mean that sportsmen and women are condemned to certain sports or activities by an 'accident of birth' because they 'chose' the wrong parents? Well, to a certain degree the answer is yes, but all is not lost. There is hope!

Recent studies have identified an **intermediate type fibre**. (Some research has suggested more, but in general they all have similar potential and can be

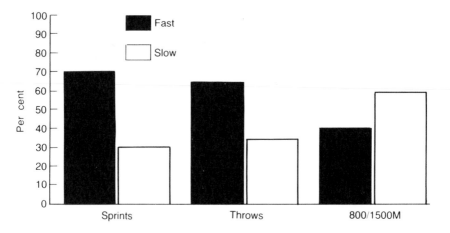

Fig. 3 *The distribution of fibre types for different activities*

put under the one heading.) This fibre possesses characteristics of both the slow and fast types, but with subtle differences. It has more endurance capacity and resistance to fatigue than a fast twitch fibre, but not as much as a red one. At the same time it contracts faster than a red fibre, but not as quickly as a white fibre.

It is thought that the intermediate fibres are more affected than the other types by the training process. For example, the sort of training which places an emphasis on stamina will develop the endurance capacity of these fibres, thereby increasing the overall ability of the muscle to tolerate such work. At the same time, speed or power training will develop the high intensity work output of the muscle. It is therefore essential that any training programme reflects the specific requirement of the chosen activity.

The coach of junior martial artists has to bear one physiological fact in mind. Until students reach the age of 16, that is when they have gone through the trauma of puberty, there is little or no fibre differentiation. It seems that the specific function of fibres is controlled by hormones which are not present until after this period. So, any extremes of speed, strength or endurance will not be possible until maturity has been reached.

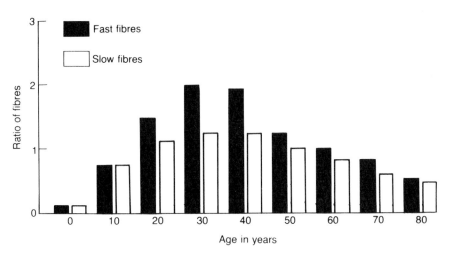

Fig. 4 *The change in fibre distribution with age*

MUSCULAR ENERGY

I have described the structure of muscles and the different qualities of the various fibre types. It is probably worth discussing at this stage how muscles produce the energy required to generate force.

Metabolism

Every cell in the body needs energy in order to perform the task for which it has been designed. This is just as true of cells making up the lungs, liver and bone as it is of muscles (obviously the requirements of muscles tend to be more dynamic and demanding than those of other tissues). Similarly, any active cell is not going to need raw materials just for energy, but for growth and repair as well. These chemical reactions which ensure both the function and continued existence of a cell are known collectively as **metabolism**.

Metabolism is made up of two elements.

Catabolism

Catabolism is the breaking-down process in the cell through which energy and materials required for the cell's function are used up.

Anabolism

Anabolism is the replenishing of energy and material stores necessary for the healthy functioning of the cell.

Metabolism, then, is the combined process of catabolism and anabolism, and at any moment in time a cell is in a dynamic state of both processes. The greater the demand placed upon a cell, the greater the rate of metabolism is to meet those increased needs. It therefore follows that at rest a student's rate of metabolism will be less than when he (and obviously the cells from which he is made) is physically active.

If we consider the specific needs of the martial arts in terms of the varied ways in which muscles are asked to function, then in reality we have to concentrate on the skeletal muscles. This doesn't mean that cardiac and smooth muscle are not as important, but within the limitations of the book there is no scope to describe their role fully.

Energy systems

With skeletal muscle there are basically two kinds of energy system.

The aerobic system

With this energy pathway all the energy production processes take place with an ample supply of oxygen. This system is usually associated with low-intensity, long-duration activity.

The anaerobic system

With this energy pathway all energy production processes take place in the absence of oxygen. The system is usually associated with high-intensity, short-duration activity.

Metabolism, then, can occur with or without oxygen. However, nutrients are essential for all processes, particularly for anabolism. These nutritional elements, along with minerals and vitamins that are essential for good health, are to be found in the foods that we eat. With respect to energy production, the three main elements of our diet are **fats, carbohydrates** and **proteins**.

	Energy in calories	Oxygen required	Carbon dioxide produced	Calories per litre of oxygen
Fat	9	2	1.5	4.5
Carbohydrate	4	1	1	3
Protein	4	1	1	4
	Per gramme	(in litres)		

The relationship between nutrients, gases and energy production (approximate values)

Fats

Theoretically, fats are the most energy-rich of the three elements. The only difficulty with their use is that they require a disproportionate amount of oxygen to produce energy. In addition, when energy is made available part of the resulting by-products are large amounts of carbon dioxide that have to be removed. This tends to identify fats as a source of energy for low-intensity, long-duration activity. Such exercise allows for an abundant supply of oxygen availability, but at the same time facilitates the removal of waste products, particularly carbon dioxide. Fats, therefore, are very much an aerobic energy source.

Proteins

Proteins demand almost as much oxygen as fats to maximise their potential, but they are a poor energy pathway. They seem to be the muscle's last option for energy generation, since actual muscle tissue may have to be broken down which may, of course, cause structural damage. Such a situation might occur when all other forms of energy-providing material are no longer present, for example in a person with a poor or reduced food intake. Similarly, the amount of waste products produced, especially carbon dioxide, is proportionally higher than that produced by a similar quantity of fat. In addition, it is not readily removed.

Carbohydrates

These probably provide the commonest energy source for students of martial arts. They yield a high level of energy for a relatively low oxygen requirement, while at the same time they produce low levels of carbon dioxide. They tend to be more suitable for intermediate and intense levels of work, preferably with oxygen, although they can still be used without. In other words, they can be broken down aerobically or anaerobically.

Fig. 5 shows the relationship between the aerobic and the anaerobic energy systems, and the different demands of the martial arts.

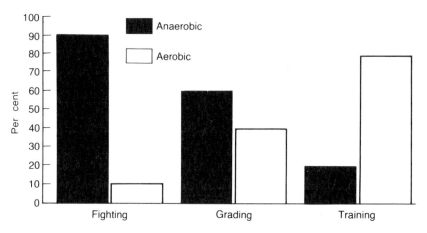

Fig. 5 *The energy demands of martial arts activities*

Energy availability

The only source of energy that cells, particularly those in muscles, use is a substance known as **adenosine triphosphate** (ATP). Fats, carbohydrates and protein are simply the fuel which is used to produce ATP in a similar way that coal, oil, wind and radioactive sources in power stations all produce the single product, electricity. It is the rate at which these 'fuels' produce ATP to 'power' muscular contraction that is the critical factor.

Fats and carbohydrates, in the form of **glycogen**, are stored in the muscle and are readily available for use. Protein, if required, usually has to come from the breakdown of cellular tissue through the process known as **catabolism**. This will naturally affect the functioning of the cell and is a last 'choice'.

ATP is stored in units called **mitochondria** which may be regarded as the batteries of the muscle cell. To continue this analogy, fats, carbohydrates and protein are the fuel for 'recharging' them.

Muscles 'prefer' to work aerobically, i.e. in the presence of oxygen, for several reasons.

1 'Fuels' produce ATP more efficiently in the presence of oxygen, and certainly for the majority of the normal demands of daily life, such as sleeping, sitting, walking, most work and school activity, this tends to be the case.

2 With the presence of oxygen, the only by-products of the process, apart from ATP, are carbon dioxide and water which the muscles' 'waste removal' systems are especially well-developed for removing. Although the muscle in particular and the body in general have stores of the main fuels – fats and carbohydrates – fatigue through physical activity usually occurs because of the build-up of waste products (and not through exhaustion of these stores).

3 With an abundant supply of oxygen, at low levels of activity muscles will tend to use fats as their first 'choice' of fuel. This is because there are large stores of fats and because carbohydrate can be 'saved' for more demanding aerobic activity.

As the intensity of work increases, carbohydrates can be broken down anaerobically, i.e. when energy demand outstrips oxygen supply. Since fats can be used as a fuel only when oxygen is present, it seems logical to protect carbohydrate stores, which are much more versatile, whenever possible.

4 Though muscles can work anaerobically, they do so inefficiently. There are problems which arise from the supply of ATP both during and after exercise.

When periods of intensive work are required of muscles, the demand for energy simply outstrips the supply of oxygen. Even when the supply is sufficient, waste products – carbon dioxide and water – are produced, although the cell is able to deal with them relatively effectively. However, without oxygen the fuels work much less efficiently and produce a more problematical waste product, **lactic acid**. It is the build-up of this product which eventually stops the energy supply in the cell, simply because it is so difficult to remove; it is a case of self-inflicted 'cellular pollution'. Incidentally, it is lactic acid that gives rise to sore and aching muscles during intensive work.

Furthermore, lactic acid requires oxygen to break it down so that it can be removed, which of course can only come about by rest or much lower levels of activity. That is why after stopping intensive exercise students still breathe rapidly and deeply to get oxygen to the cells to break down the acid into more easily handled waste. The amount of time it takes heart rate and breathing to return to normal will depend upon the levels of lactic acid present and the amount of oxygen required to process it. The situation is known as **repaying the oxygen debt**. Fig. 6 shows the relationship between the demand for ATP and the presence or lack of oxygen.

Energy pathways

Anaerobic (without oxygen)

Anaerobic
alactic
(no lactate)

$$ATP \longrightarrow ADP + P + Energy$$
(This system lasts for only 2–3 seconds.)

$$ADP + PC \longrightarrow ATP + Creatine$$

(Phosphero-creatine is stored in the muscle cell. There is 3 times more PC than ATP. This system lasts for 10–15 seconds.)

Anaerobic
lactic
(lactate
produced)

$$Glycogen + P + ADP \underline{\hspace{1cm}} ATP + Lactate$$
(Glycogen is broken down in the absence of oxygen.
This system lasts for 45–60 seconds at 100% effort until exhaustion.)

Aerobic (with oxygen)

$$Glycogen + P + ADP + Oxygen \longrightarrow ATP + Carbon + Water$$
1 unit $\quad\quad\quad\quad\quad\quad\quad\quad\quad\quad\quad$ 37 $\quad$ Dioxide
units
energy

$$Fats + P + ADP + Oxygen \longrightarrow ATP + Carbon + Water$$
1 unit $\quad\quad\quad\quad\quad\quad\quad\quad\quad\quad\quad$ 140 $\quad$ Dioxide
units
energy

(These systems are capable of periods of prolonged activity at low intensity.)

Fig. 6 *The production of energy for the martial arts*

As ATP is being used during low levels of muscular activity, it is readily replaced by the combined efforts of fats and oxygen. However, if there is a sudden and intense demand for energy, several systems swing into action. For ATP to release its stored energy it has to be broken down into **adenosine diphosphate** (ADP) and a 'broken off' **phosphate**. In fact, it is the 'break' which releases the energy. To recharge the mitochondria the two have to be recombined so that they can 'break' again when required.

In the very short term of 2–3 seconds, all energy demands can be met by stores of ATP in the mitochondria. If an intense demand continues, the stores of **phosphero creatine** (PC) are utilised as a means of recycling 'used' ATP (transformed into ADP and a P, and then back into ATP again to provide more energy). The advantage of this system is that the waste products from the breakdown of ATP combine with PC to produce more ATP without any further waste products such as lactic acid. The processes are referred to as **anaerobic alactic systems**.

Eventually, after about 10–15 seconds the PC system runs down. If there is still a demand for energy, it can only be satisfied by drawing upon reserves of glycogen. Since the demand is so intense and there is not sufficient time to circulate oxygen, the muscles will be working anaerobically. Glycogen, therefore, provides the fuel to recombine the ADP and the free P. ATP is produced without the presence of oxygen, but so is lactic acid. This pathway is brought to a halt by the presence of the lactate after 45–60 seconds. The energy system is known as the Anaerobic Lactic System.

If the demand for energy continues, then by this time oxygen can be brought to active tissue. In such a situation any waste products are carbon dioxide and water which can be removed fairly easily. If muscular energy has to be sustained in relatively low levels of intensity, once again fats and carbohydrates can be used as the fuel for ATP synthesis.

Role of the fibre types

When looking at the energy pathways for muscular activity the role of the different fibre types has to be considered since each has particular qualities (see Fig. 7).

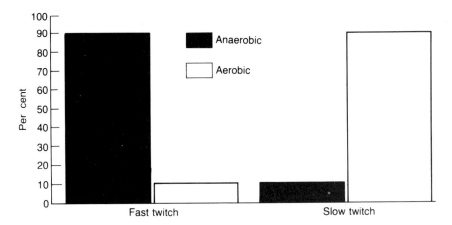

Fig. 7 *The relationship between energy production and fibre types*

Slow twitch fibres

These have a rich blood supply which is designed to supply oxygen. They will predominantly be used for low levels of activity, with fats in the first instance as the fuel source. As the level for energy increases, the fuel source will switch to carbohydrate since it requires less oxygen for a given workload.

Fast twitch fibres

These do not have a well-developed blood supply system and so are better designed for anaerobic work. Stores of phosphero creatine and the fibres' ability to use glycogen without oxygen allow for short periods of intense activity before waste products build up.

Intermediate fibres

As previously identified, these have characteristics of both types. They tend to use glycogen aerobically for periods of long duration and low energy output, or anaerobically for short, intensive periods.

So, the picture seems to be that slow twitch fibres are normally used; as the load increases, intermediate ones are recruited until, finally, for maximal effort, fast twitch fibres are called upon (see Fig. 8).

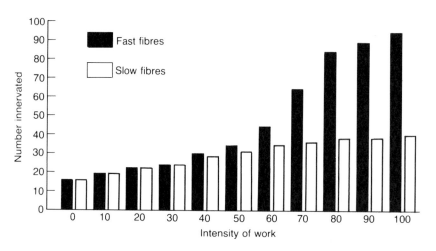

Fig. 8 *The number of muscle fibres required to overcome resistance*

TYPES OF STRENGTH

In the martial arts there is such a wide range of activities that to identify a specific type of strength is impossible. For example, what are the similarities between tai chi and full-contact competitions? I would suggest very little, since each has its own specific requirements. Perhaps it might be useful if the term 'strength' were developed with the help of a few definitions.

Strength

Strength can be defined as the tension or force that a muscle or group of muscles can exert against a resistance.

The definition simply explains that muscles contract to generate force, but what help is this in identifying the needs of martial arts?

Maximum or absolute strength

This is the greatest tension or force that the **neuro-muscular system** is capable of generating in one conscious effort.

How many martial arts skills are performed just once with *maximum* effort? Possibly only those that involve such activities as breaking techniques.

Relative strength or strength to weight ratio

This is the greatest tension or force that the muscular system can exert as a proportion of body weight.

$$\frac{\text{relative}}{\text{strength}} = \frac{\text{maximum strength}}{\text{body weight}}$$

Here it is not the actual force generated or weight lifted which is critical but how it compares with the student's own body weight. For example, one student weighs 75 kg (165 lb) and 'dead lifts' 150 kg (330 lb), and another student weighs 100 kg (220 lb) and performs the same lift. Both have managed to lift the same weight, but the first student has lifted twice his body weight while the second managed only one and a half times his. Despite the fact that both students have managed the same weight, the first is obviously the stronger of the two. When the weight lifted is compared to body weight, most martial arts are concerned with the ability of a student to handle his own body weight, so perhaps this aspect of strength is important.

Plyometric or elastic strength

This is the ability of the muscles to act explosively.

After technique, most martial artists would suggest that being able to perform at speed is very important. I suppose the concept of 'power' is embraced by this type of muscle action.

Strength endurance

A suitable definition would be: the ability of the muscles to generate force in an ever-increasing climate of fatigue.

Being able to withstand the repetition of techniques in a lesson, or being able to reproduce techniques over a period of time in gradings and competition, is an essential element of the martial arts.

Local muscular endurance

This is the ability of muscles to generate force in an ever-increasing climate of fatigue at a local level.

For example, in developing strength endurance in, say, punching techniques, the student is limited by fatigue developing in the upper body. In the main, the other muscles are not being stressed to the same levels, so if the arms had more tolerance to fatigue, the student could work longer.

Will-power

The ability of a student to concentrate on the maximum voluntary effort needed to achieve maximum/optimum strength constitutes will-power.

This really is the intangible element in all training. It is suggested that at best we are only able consciously to generate about 20% of our maximum strength. In cases of extreme emotional or psychological stress these 'safety mechanisms' are over-ridden and feats of phenomenal strength have been noted. If a student can tap those resources, performance at any level will be improved.

Joint movement

Strength, or its application, depends to a large extent upon the range of movement through which the joint (or the muscle which controls the range of movement) acts. It might be helpful if the movement at a joint is described.

Full range of movement occurs when a muscle contracts from its maximum normal length to its shortest contracted state, thus moving a joint through its greatest possible range.

The biceps curl in an excellent example of the range through which a limb, and the weight being lifted, can be moved.

The full range of movement at a joint can be divided into three sections. The **outer range** is the angle through which the muscle, at its maximum length,

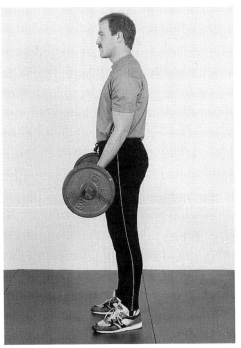

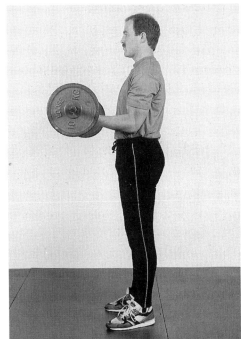

Above left *The biceps curl. The exercise begins in the outer movement range of the elbow joint*

Above right *Midway through the elbows' range of movement*

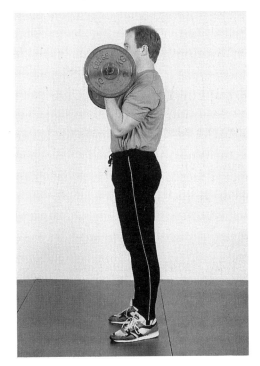

At this point in the exercise the biceps muscles are at their shortest length and the elbows are moving in the inner range

acts on a joint. The **mid range** occurs towards the middle point of the contraction and range of movement at a joint. The **inner range** occurs from the mid range towards the shortest possible length of the muscle.

The action of a joint and its associated muscles is worthy of far more than academic interest. Because of the mechanical principles involved, the weight to be lifted or the force to be generated will be dependent upon the range through which it is to be moved.

In the outer range, because of the long levers involved, muscles are not very efficient. Therefore, the load they can lift or the force which they can generate will be limited. As the movement approaches the mid-point, muscles become more efficient and consequently the force which they generate is greater. As the action continues, from the mid to the inner range, the force generated is at its greatest.

In general, the problem is that only a light weight can be used in the outer range. So, as the action continues and the muscles work more efficiently, they are not being worked to their maximum potential. In an attempt to overcome this mechanical problem and the disadvantages of the outer range, many weight lifters cheat by jerking or swinging the weights at the start of the movement. This allows them to use a sufficient load to work the muscles intensively in the mid and inner ranges.

Function of muscles

Although it clearly can be seen that there are several 'types' of strength, the picture is made cloudier if one looks at the way in which muscles function. The simple notion that they only contract or shorten to produce the desired result is no longer completely valid. Broadly speaking, four types of muscle action or strength have been identified.

Isotonic strength

The muscle shortens through the entire range of movement, because the force it can generate is greater than the resistance against which it is working.

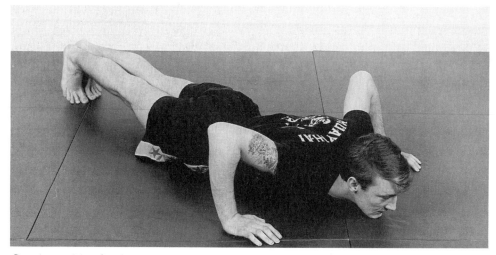

Starting position for the press-up

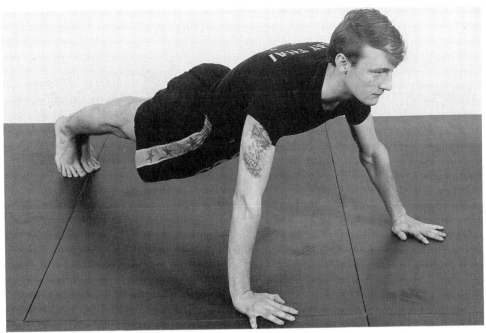

The student thrusts upwards with his arms, thereby contracting his triceps muscles

The classic press-up is a typical example of isotonic muscle action. The photograph on page 24 shows the starting position of the exercise. The triceps, that is the muscles at the back of the upper arm, are fully stretched, initially working in the outer range. They shorten through their full range to straighten the arm (see the photograph above).

Isometric strength

The muscle does not change in length, since the force it generates is equal to the resistance against which it is working. Sometimes this type of muscle action is also known as **static strength**.

A typical example of an isometric contraction is illustrated. The student attempts a normal press-up, while a partner stops the movement by holding the shoulders. Although the student continues to push as hard as possible, the triceps do not shorten any further. The practical problem with this type of activity is that muscles are only worked maximally in part of the movement range. The situation can be resolved by practising isometric contractions at different positions (see photographs overleaf).

Isokinetic strength

The muscle shortens in length while at the same time working at maximum throughout the entire range of movement.

Very expensive items of equipment are available to develop isokinetic strength; however, a partner can be just as effective. For example, a partner

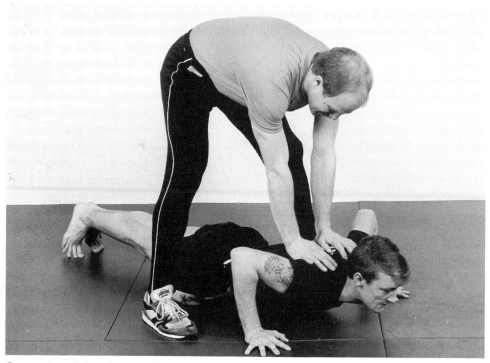

Contraction of the triceps muscles held in the outer range

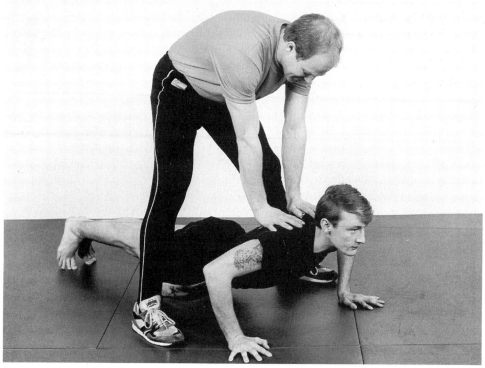

Contraction held in the mid range

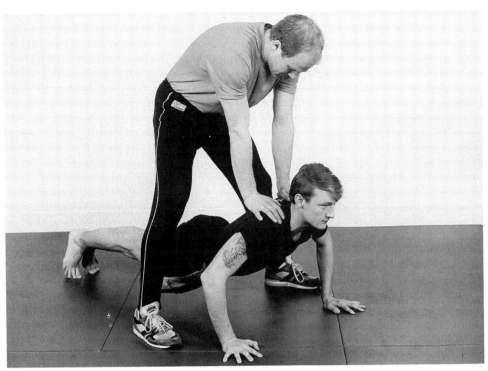

Triceps contraction held in the mid to inner range

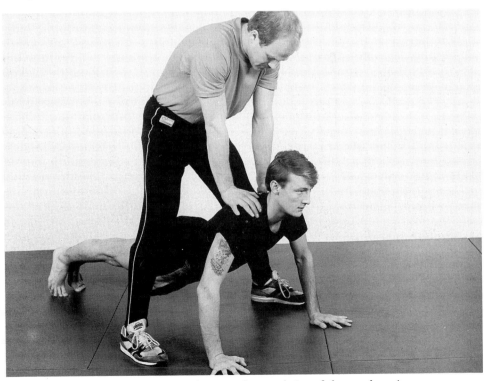

Contraction held in the inner range, almost at the completion of the muscle action

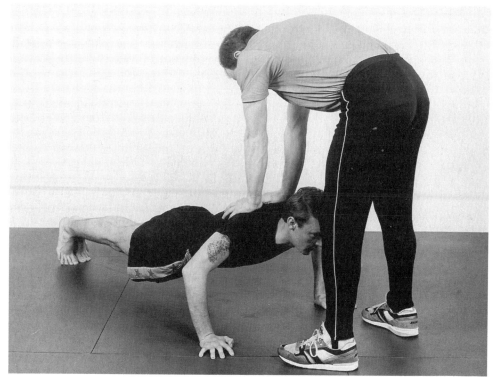

A partner is helping a student to develop isokinetic strength by applying pressure to his shoulders. The student presses against the resistance

holds down the shoulders as a student attempts a press-up. The partner changes the resistance throughout the entire range of movement. In the early stages of the action, when the triceps are working in their outer range and therefore not very efficiently, he does not have to apply much effort. However, as the action continues, he will have to hold the shoulders down with ever-increasing force as the muscles involved become progressively more efficient. There should be no pause in the press-up action; the movement should be continuous. The speed of the action is controlled by the changing resistance of the partner.

Plyometric strength

The muscle lengthens or stretches under a load, and then contracts very quickly. This pre-stretched muscle, like a stretched elastic band, will contract faster and more powerfully than in a normal contraction.

In this example of the press-up a partner acts as a support. The student slowly lowers himself towards his partner's back. The use of a partner in this way obviously reduces the load on the shoulders by placing more weight upon the feet. When the student's chest just touches his partner's back he pushes up as fast and as hard as possible.

The triceps are slowly stretched as the student lowers himself. However, they are also in a state of semi-contraction because they are controlling the rate of descent. Since the muscles are stretched and already partially contracted, when they are required to contract fully they will do so faster and with greater force than if they were in a relaxed state.

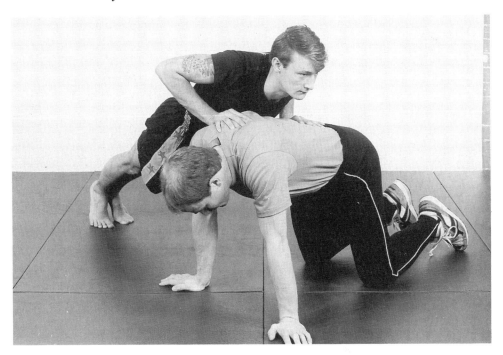

A partner helps a student to develop plyometric strength

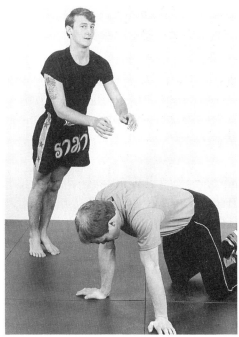

The student pushes up quickly from the press-up position

THE EFFECT OF TRAINING

As we have seen, the demands of the different martial arts are very specific. The coach has to identify the type of strength which has particular style requires. However, whichever aspect is wanted, each is acquired through the common principle of **overload**.

For any strength training programme to be successful a muscle, or group of muscles, has to be worked at intensities which are not normally dealt with. The body responds to being stressed or overloaded beyond normal everyday requirements by adapting the tissues involved to tolerate the new demands. So, strength work has to stress muscles appropriately for them to become stronger and able to cope with the greater workload.

Once the muscles have adapted, then the load must be made even greater for them to increase further in strength. This is where **strength training** is probably better described as **progressive resistance training**. Muscles adapt to cope with a particular load and they will maintain that strength level until the workload is increased once again. Therefore, loadings have to be systematically and progressively increased as muscles develop strength.

How muscles adapt will depend on the type of strength required, and any adaptation will take into account the development of the types of muscle fibre involved. Short-term intense activity will develop the *fast twitch fibres* and will modify the *intermediate fibres* to work in a similar way, while long-term endurance activity will tend to develop the *slow twitch fibres* and will modify the *intermediate fibres* to work in a comparable fashion. It can be seen, then, that because muscles adapt specifically to the type of work to which they are subjected, the exact demands of each martial art have to be identified and trained for accordingly. Put simply: training must reflect the needs of the activity or technique.

The difficulty with strength training is that it usually is seen as either weight or circuit training. This is far from the reality of the situation. Strength can be developed by using:

- body weight
- barbells
- dumb-bells
- ankle weights
- wrist weights
- multi-gyms
- nautilus machines

- medicine balls
- lifting stones
- lifting logs
- sand bags
- weighted jackets
- springs
- elastic ropes

- bullworkers
- pulleys
- ropes
- running up steps
- running up hills
- running in sand
- running in heavy boots
- running in surf
- running, towing a tyre
- gymnasium equipment.

Very often these forms of strength training are much better suited than the traditional weight and circuit training to the needs of martial artists. In addition, with a little imagination, strength training activities can be devised which are not only specific to a particular martial art, but which mirror the exact techniques used (see examples later in the book).

SYSTEMS OF TRAINING

In order for the coach to devise training programmes which are going to meet the needs of his students, he must understand their construction. From the instantaneous production of strength for breaking techniques to the demands of arduous grading, competition and training, schedules can be devised to produce the desired results. As we have seen, training brings about very specific adaptations of the tissues to the type of work to which they are subjected. It is essential, therefore, that the coach and the student get the training right. It takes a long time for changes to occur – weeks, months and, more likely, years – so any training errors will take a long time to correct.

It does not matter which sort of resistance the student uses; the same principles apply. However, certain types of equipment will favour the development of particular aspects of strength. With any training programme the coach must consider:

- **intensity**: the degree to which muscles are worked
- **duration**: how long the muscles are subjected to the workload
- **frequency**: how often the muscles are subjected to the workload.

In practical terms this usually means the following. 'Intensity' is normally referred to as the **load**, which is the weight or resistance against which the muscles are working. 'Duration' can be the number of **repetitions** of a particular activity, or a period of **time** in which to perform a given number of repetitions or as many repetitions as possible. 'Frequency' is a recommended number of **sets** of repetitions.

Designing programmes

The permutations of **intensity/load, duration/repetitions** and **frequency/sets** give the coach the ability to create training regimes which will bring about specific types of strength. The following examples might be a guideline to the preparation of such programmes of work based upon 'types' of strength.

To design such programmes a student's maximum work rate (i.e. the maximum load or number of repetitions that he can perform) should be ascertained through carefully arranged sessions. The examples shown are

Type of strength	Load in % of max.	Possible repetitions	Possible sets
Maximum strength	95	3	3
	90	4	3
	85	6	3
General strength	75	8	3
	70	10	3
Strength endurance	65	12	3
	60	15	3
Local muscular endurance	50	20	3
	40	25	3
	30	30	3
Plyometric strength	30	6–10	3
	40	3–9	3
Power	10–25	6–10	3
Speed	5–10	6–10	3

Fig. 9 *Weight training systems and strength development*

based on the premiss that the coach knows what the student's maximum work rate is in each activity concerned.

Fig. 9 illustrates the relationship between the workload and the number of repetitions.

Maximum or absolute strength

To develop this type of strength the muscles have to be worked to maximum or near maximum levels, but only two or three times in a short period because the demands placed on muscle fibre and energy systems are enormous.

Typical systems are:

- 3 sets of 3 repetitions at 95% of maximum
- 3 sets of 4 repetitions at 90% of maximum
- 3 sets of 6 repetitions at 85% of maximum.

The intensity of the load varies slightly, but the training effect is maintained by increasing the number of repetitions. 'Pyramid systems' might be included for the advanced student. These could be as follows:

- 5 repetitions at 80%
- 4 repetitions at 85%
- 3 repetitions at 90%
- 2 repetitions at 95%
- 1 repetition at 100%.

With this system, the number of repetitions is decreased as the load is increased. When the student reaches one repetition, he can try a heavier weight than his previous best and can keep going until he is unable to lift any further. A variation is to work from 5–1 and then back down again from 1–5. For maximal efforts the system might be varied to:

- 3 repetitions at 90%
- 2 repetitions at 95%
- 1 repetition at 100%.
- The single lift should be repeated until the student fails.

General strength

If a student has to be able to perform a strength-demanding activity several times for his martial art, the number of repetitions should be increased. However, remember that the load should also be reduced.

Typical systems might be:

- 3 sets of 8 repetitions at 75%
- 3 sets of 10 repetitions at 70%.

When a student needs to perform an action repeatedly, the emphasis shifts from **absolute strength** to **strength endurance**. This is achieved quite easily by increasing the number of repetitions and by reducing the load.

Such systems might be:

- 3 sets of 12 repetitions at 65%
- 4 sets of 15 repetitions at 60%.

However, if more stamina is required, then the duration of the effort has to be increased at the expense of the load. This leads to **local muscular endurance** where normally the student is handling only his body weight.

Such a system might be:

- 3 sets of 30 repetitions at 30%.

Rather than work simply for repetitions as a variant, the student can attempt to perform as many actions as possible in a given time. For example:

- 3 sets of 30 seconds of continuous work.

The time period can be extended to match the time constraint of a competition, e.g. for as long as 2 or 3 minutes, or it can be shortened to match periods of intense activity, e.g. 10–20 seconds.

Isometric strength

This type of strength is identified by a muscle 'holding' a position without movement. The sort of activity is characterised by muscles being contracted to maximum without them changing in length.

Typical training might be:

- holding a maximum contraction for 5–9 seconds; this could be repeated 5–8 times, with 2–3 sets.

Isometric contraction only works a muscle to maximum at one point in the entire range of movement. There is a much better way of utilising this type of muscular activity. Select an action in which the above example of a training load can be executed at four points, from the outer range to the fully contracted state. A suitable programme would be:

- 4–6 (depending on the number of points in the range of movement) sets of 5–8 maximum-effort contractions, each held for 5–9 seconds.

Plyometric strength

Such strength development requires the muscles to contract maximally and explosively. The only way that this can happen is if the load is light, usually body weight or less. The muscles also have to be 'pre-stretched' prior to contraction. The analogy of the elastic band may again be helpful: a band shortens much faster if it is stretched to its maximum length before being allowed to contract.

Since plyometric strength training is very demanding on muscles, tendons and the nervous system, repetitions need to be monitored carefully.

Possible systems might be:

- 3 sets of 6–10 repetitions with a light load, 10–20%
- 3 sets of 3–6 repetitions with a heavy load, 40% – body weight.

Speed Any movements at high speed demand a great effort from the muscles involved. Research in Germany seems to suggest that speed can be developed, but that the loads must not exceed 5–10% of maximum. If the load exceeds this amount, then speed is sacrificed for strength.

Such systems might be:

- 3 sets of 6–10 repetitions at 5–10% of maximum.

Power Since this type of muscle action tends to be a compromise between strength and speed, loads need to be light and the action must be performed at maximum speed. Great care should be taken, because any load moving at speed could pose great structural danger to joints and connective tissue.

A typical system might be:

- 3 sets of 6–10 repetitions at 10–25% of maximum.

Rest With all the programmes described, there has to be sufficient time for recovery between sets. The coach and the student have to decide between them what is an appropriate rest to allow for the successful completion of an exercise or programme.

Further considerations

Fig. 10 shows the relationship between the load and the speed of movement; it is usually referred to as the 'force-velocity' curve. Basically, it identifies the fact that a heavy load cannot be moved quickly, whereas a light one can be! It really

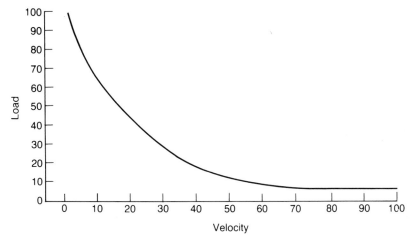

Fig. 10 *The relationship between the load lifted and the speed of development*

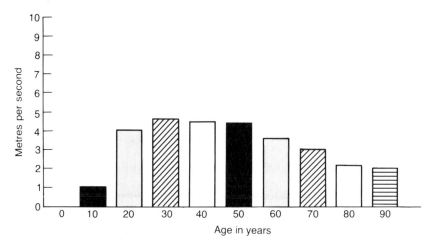

Fig. 11 *The relationship between limb speed and age*

confirms the relationship between loads, repetitions and the development of various types of strength.

This state of affairs is unfortunately modified by other factors such as age and fibre type. Fig. 11 shows how limb speed varies with age. Speed levels, as an indication of strength, will increase with maturation to peak at the age

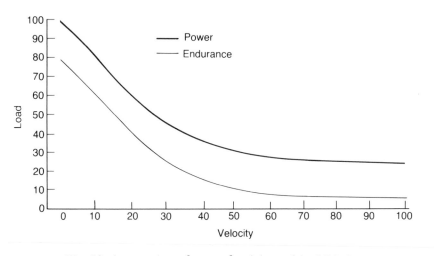

Fig. 12 *A comparison of types of activity and load lifted*

of approximately 25 years. Fig. 12 identifies how fibre distribution in sportsmen and women, categorised by endurance or power, affects work output at all points. The endurance athletes produce less power with any load than the power group.

STRENGTH TRAINING PROGRAMMES

Some of the more academic and practical aspects of strength training have now been identified. Once the coach has decided what type of strength a student needs to develop, he can devise appropriate combinations of loads, repetitions and sets. However, that is only part of the picture. There are further considerations: for example, which exercises should be chosen?; how many exercises should a coach include in a student's schedule?

Over many years of designing strength training programmes I have evolved the following 'formula' to help in structuring programmes. I divide all exercises into four broad categories:

- **upper body** – neck, shoulders and arms
- **trunk** – abdominals and lower back
- **legs** – thighs and lower legs
- **general** – exercises which involve most of the muscle groups.

Example of a strength training programme

A typical programme would be:

1 an arm exercise
2 an abdominal exercise
3 a thigh exercise
4 a whole body exercise
5 a shoulder exercise
6 a lower back exercise
7 a calf exercise
8 a whole body exercise.

In a normal programme I would select eight exercises (two from each of the four categories), and I would tend to follow the above pattern. The first exercise is aimed at developing strength in the arms so that by the time the activity has been completed they are tired! While they are recovering another muscle group can be exercised, in this case the abdominals. While the abdominals and the arms continue to recover, the thighs can be worked. In turn, while the thighs, as well as the abdominals and arms, recover a general whole body exercise can be performed. After this the arms will have rested sufficiently to perform another exercise but using a different group of muscles. Then the abdominals and lower back can be worked, and so on. Put simply, work one group of muscles while others rest and recover. Of course this is only successful if the exercises use different parts of the body; for example, two arm exercises in succession would not, for the average student, be a good idea.

As I pointed out earlier, a typical strength training programme might consist of a balanced combination of eight exercises. However, should a coach recognise that a student has a weakness or a specific need, perhaps in the requirements for an advanced technique, emphasis could be placed on a particular part of the body or type of strength. In such a situation a coach might identify 10 or 12 exercises which include a number of specific movements for meeting the student's needs.

There is a further aspect, that of mixing the training regimes, which the coach might want to bear in mind. There is no reason why every exercise should follow the same system of load, repetitions and sets. For example, a coach might want to develop explosive power in the arms and legs at the same time as isometric strength in the back and abdominal muscles.

TRAINING REQUIREMENTS

The concept of strength training for the martial arts immediately poses the difficulty of each discipline and style having its own specific requirements. With this fact in mind it might be useful to look at the different strength needs of some of the martial arts.

Karate

If one takes numbers of students as being the measure of success, then karate is probably the most popular martial art. It has a long history and lends itself particularly well to illustrating both the development of and the general requirements for a martial art. If the breakdown of age group ratios is also taken into account, karate seems to attract by far and away the greatest number of juniors, i.e. students under the age of 16. The training requirements and limitations of juniors must be identified; it is essential that all training, especially exercises designed to improve strength, take these points into account.

It has to be accepted that karate is based on impact-type activities, such as kicks and punches, and so aspects of strength are an intrinsic part of almost all techniques. Students, especially those who are physically immature, must take care to avoid damage to hands and feet caused by contact with hard surfaces. Indeed, all training for juniors has to be carefully monitored to ensure that problems do not develop. Any attempt to improve technique by 'strengthening' the feet and the hands using pads, makiwara or finger-tip and knuckle press-ups should be discouraged. In all sparring activities full protective padding must be worn to prevent injury. Similarly, breaking techniques or full contact fighting can pose real dangers and should be approached with extreme caution.

It would be relatively easy to explain the strength requirements for karate, but for the fact that there are many styles, each emphasising a particular aspect of fitness. Though everyone would probably say that the mastery of technique is the most important factor, how this is put into practice varies. Some forms identify mobility and great ranges of movement as being paramount, while others work on the development of speed, and yet others on strength.

The difficulty of identifying the exact type of strength required is made more complicated when it is understood that most styles have a 'hard' and a 'soft' form. In addition, the teacher will be influenced by individual experiences and will have a personal preference for a particular approach to the building of strength.

During the historical development of karate and most of the other Oriental martial arts special strength-developing aids were devised. Some of the more popular items of equipment are worth studying, because they are as useful today as they were centuries ago.

Kame

Jars filled with sand or stones, known as kame, have been used to develop finger, hand, arm and shoulder strength. The student grips the jar around its neck, with the fingers spread, and lifts it from the ground. Arm and upper body strength are developed isotonically as the jar is lifted and isometrically when it is held out parallel to the floor. When kame are used in conjunction with stances, leg strength is also developed. They were and still are a very versatile and effective form of specific strength training.

Shi ishi

Shi ishi evolved as a 'one-sided dumb-bell'. A short wooden or bamboo handle is attached to a heavy stone or weight. While the student is in a specific stance the shi ishi is lifted by the handle to arm's length, parallel to the floor, and it is rotated so that the weight points upwards. It can also be swung about the shoulders, very much in the style of 'Indian clubs', or it can be used to mirror the actions of weapons training. Such traditional martial arts practices have much to recommend them because they do not require heavy loads and they use muscle groups in a similar way to actual techniques.

Tan

The tan is very similar to a weightlifting barbell. It can be a single iron bar or a length of wood or metal with fixed weights at each end. The variety of exercises which can be performed with such an item of equipment is exactly the same as that for 'free weights'.

Kongoken

This is a solid iron hoop weighing in the region of 50 kg (110 lb) that can be used to develop both specific strength and general strength in exercises mirroring fighting techniques or those of 'free weights'.

Weights

Traditionally, most martial arts have used some form of wrist and ankle weights, often in the form of iron bands. These can vary in weight and the student can have as many or as few as is required to develop the type of strength needed. The advantage of this practice is that techniques are repeated using hands and feet in the exact movement pattern required for a particular karate style.

Styles of karate

Although, arguably, Japanese in origin, many karate styles evolved elsewhere in the Orient. The most important ones traditionally are worthy of a closer study.

Gojo ryu

Gojo ryu in its 'hard' form emphasises the development of strength. Special exercises and sanchin katas, which have evolved to build strength, are an integral part of lessons. 'Soft' forms of gojo ryu seem to be taught once the harder forms have been mastered.

Uechi ryu

Uechi ryu is another style which highlights the development of strength as an intrinsic part of technique. It also develops or 'strengthens' the capacity of vital areas of the body to withstand pain.

Shotokan

Shotokan does not see the development of strength as an end in itself, but as an aid to achieve powerful kicks and punches. Training is geared towards the application of force at speed. Though specific strengthening exercises are used, the emphasis on them is not as great as it is in Goju ryu.

Shotokai

Out of shotokan evolved shotokai whose techniques rely very much on the development of speed. Training improves relaxation or a lack of tension in techniques so that both range and speed of movement are increased.

Shito ryu

Shito ryu develops power on impact as opposed to specific techniques requiring great strength.

Wado ryu

Wado ryu techniques and training are directed towards agility, mobility and speed of movement. The main theme of this style is to use the attacker's strength against him and as such there is no need for great personal power. Therefore, training tends to emphasise technique and agility rather than the generation of maximum strength.

Karate as sport

Historically, karate evolved from a need for effective fighting techniques. However, over a period of time some of the militaristic and philosophical origins have been overshadowed by a much more sport-oriented activity.

Traditionally, karate (and most other martial arts) involves students training in class lines. This poses no problems when the aim is to develop both technique and excellence of movement. Strength comes through the repetition of the activity: a technique might be repeated many times, and so strength endurance is improved. As a safety point, it should be noted that care must be taken not to lock out the arms and knees with force, because this puts tremendous loadings on the joints. The practice of sanchin katas, in which great emphasis is placed on maintaining a state of maximum tension in the muscles, is probably one of the best strength training methods for karate.

Since lessons can last up to two hours, there is a need for strength endurance so that students can practise for the entire period (this holds true for most other martial arts). There will be periods of intensive training when maximum, plyometric and relative strength are required, for example when using punch and kick pads, or when sparring. Therefore, when designing a lesson, the coach must allow for periods of high intensity work to be interspersed with less strenuous activity so that students are able to recover. He should also be especially aware that young martial artists cannot keep up sustained periods of maximum strength production and should adapt their training accordingly. The implication for their lesson is that only brief bursts of maximum effort should be requested and these should be punctuated with long periods of rest.

Karate relies predominantly on explosive, powerful action in both the legs and arms. For all students such activity is bound to place tremendous loadings on muscle, tendons and ligaments, bones and joints, which could be potentially very dangerous. The effectiveness of correct technique is a result of adaptations in strength, speed, power and skill and, in the young student, skeletal growth and development.

Jiu jitsu

Historically, jiu jitsu was a highly effective martial art and some consider it is the model from which many current styles have developed, particularly the Olympic sport of judo. There is much less emphasis on impact techniques than in karate. In fact, translated from the Japanese, *ju jitsu* means 'the gentle way'; this would seem to reinforce the idea that, though very effective, it does not require extreme development of strength and all-round fitness for a student to become accomplished.

Punching and kicking skills are part of the syllabus, but greater attention is paid to defence or restraint techniques, such as blocks and locks. The aim of training is to enable a student to defend himself against attack by using the force of the assault against the perpetrator.

In essence, jiu jitsu emphasises a continuous series of techniques in which the effort is geared towards controlling an attacker rather than punching or kicking him. This reduces the need for strength training during the course of a normal lesson. Again, the practice of katas is very helpful for the young student who will face the same problems of injury to joints and connective tissues as the karateka does. Although impact injuries are less of a problem than in karate, care must be taken when applying locks. Immature joints are particularly vulnerable and may be easily damaged. Part of the training process should be to strengthen them by developing the surrounding musculature at the same time as improving the range of movement. Applying and withstanding locking and blocking techniques, if practised properly, can be most beneficial in this respect.

Some skills are taught in the same way as for karate, i.e. in rank and file. However, most training involves students working in pairs. They take it in turns to practise the application of techniques. The work load generally requires strength endurance, but occasionally very intensive activity is called for when plyometric rather than maximum strength is needed. The coach should be aware of these aspects when planning lessons.

The main difference between karate and jiu jitsu is in the emphasis on speed. Karate tends to isolate limb speed, and favours the fast kick or punch. Although limb speed is still of importance in jiu jitsu, whole body speed or agility is the key factor. Students require more in the way of elastic strength and mobility. Since there is no need to develop maximum strength, loadings on joints and connective tissue will be much reduced. By being less demanding physically than karate, ju jitsu is a very popular martial art with students of all ages and both sexes.

Judo

Judo as both an 'art' and a 'sport' focuses initially on wrestling-type activities by means of which a judoka tries to find an advantage so he can trip, throw, lock or hold down his opponent. Although general strength is vital, because all parts of the body are involved in any technique, development of the arms, upper torso and legs is important.

It is quite clear that judo has its roots in ju jitsu from which it evolved as a 'softer' form. At the highest levels it is intensive and demanding, especially in competition, but for the young and the less committed martial artist it need not be so. Normally practice is in pairs, with the students taking it in turns to apply a technique. Since there is no punching or kicking, danger to the judo student is less than for the karateka, but the use of locks has to be carefully controlled.

In 'traditional' judo there were many katas which are generally not taught today but which would be an invaluable part of lessons for the development of specific strength. At first there is a need for endurance to allow a student to throw and apply techniques for the duration of the lesson. As techniques develop, there is a much greater demand for periods of intense activity in which skills are applied with speed. These require plyometric strength.

Due to the number of throwing and take-down techniques employed in judo, it is vital that breakfalls are fully covered in the initial development of skills. Falling backwards, sideways and forwards in an ineffective manner can overload very vulnerable parts of the body; this identifies a need for agility in all breakfall techniques. Relative strength, or the sort of strength that gymnasts build, is obviously a very important element in the training programme.

Aikido

Traditionally, aikido involves little in the way of explosive action. This seems to be contradictory to the needs of the competitive side of the activity. As with jiu jitsu, whole body speed or agility is more important than limb speed, so the development of maximum strength has no place in the training programme. Aikido utilises the opponent's force and aggression against him. It is manifestly defensive, not offensive, in nature.

The emphasis seems to be on the use of a series of techniques which depend on skill rather than on effort. Therefore, the development of strength seems to go against the philosophy of the discipline. Training identifies psychological rather than physical components; it could be viewed as a martial arts contest of wits! This aspect could be borne in mind by the other martial arts, since it makes aikido an attractive activity to students of all ages and levels of fitness.

Training is normally conducted with students in pairs, each taking turns to apply techniques, thereby allowing for a recovery between periods of semi-intensive activity.

Although a general level of basic strength is ideal, there is no need to train to extremes. Endurance in general and plyometric strength in particular are the main requirements. Perhaps educating the body to be flexible 'with strength' might be the best way to sum up part of an aikido practitioner's aim.

Hapkido

Hapkido seems to combine the punches and kicks of karate with the wrestling and throwing techniques of ju jitsu, judo and aikido. Execution of good and appropriate technique, rather than using 'brute force', is important. The sort of strength required would appear to be a combination of all styles, which poses a very difficult problem for the coach to resolve! The possible dangers of impact techniques associated with karate and of locks and blocks with jiu jitsu have to be considered.

Once again, the teaching styles of hapkido are very similar to those of karate and ju jitsu, students training in rank and file and also practising kata and partner work.

Kendo

Kendo is an impact-based activity in which the force generated is transmitted to the opponent by a bamboo sword or shinai. Any potential dangers to the combatants are very much reduced by a comprehensive set of armour covering the entire body, especially the head.

The need for strength lies in the application of technique, though purists might argue that correct state of mind is of greater importance. Strength endurance, particularly in the upper body, has to be developed not only to withstand the rigours of the lesson but also to cope with the additional resistance of the protective armour. Techniques, as in most martial arts, require elastic strength to help generate powerful movements in a very short period of time. Training tends to be dominated by sparring, but an element of class activity and katas seems well suited to the development of the strength requirements of most students.

Kung fu

The definition of kung fu as a martial art presents many difficulties. There are a number of different 'styles' and 'family interpretations' which make it almost impossible to identify common requirements for training, grading and competition. The position is made even more difficult by the concept of 'hard' and 'soft' forms.

The main part of all types of kung fu, however, seems to be the application of inner energy or chi. The refinement of specific types of strength, therefore, seems to be less important than the development of techniques and the correct state of mind. Though punches and kicks are an element of training, they are performed in a relaxed manner without too much emphasis on speed or strength. So, the development of elastic strength seems to be essential. Wooden mannequins are a traditional form of training designed to 'strengthen' hands, forearms and legs. However, their use probably desensitises the body to pain rather than strengthens muscles.

Under the 'umbrella' title of kung fu, tai chi has a very important role. With this martial art, perhaps more than with any other, the emphasis is on relaxation and form. The extensive use of both long and short form katas can only add to its benefits for the students of all ages and abilities, since underdeveloped body systems are not being overloaded. Class drills and sparring form the major components of lessons.

Shorinji kempo

Shorinji kempo has a very similar strength requirement to hapkido and, as might be expected, training follows a similar pattern. Emphasis is laid on the philosophical and psychological approach to the activity, as well as on the development of a correct attitude and state of mind for the application of techniques and training. Self-discipline in training, grading and competition is essential and any specific strength development is subordinate to the appropriate application of technique.

Tang soo do

The specific strength requirements of tang soo do are very similar to those of karate, but perhaps more attention is given to higher kicking techniques, like those in taekwando. There is therefore a need to develop the explosive plyometric strength of the legs. Training tends to follow a very similar pattern to that of karate.

Taekwando

Taekwando training resembles that of tang soo do and karate, except that there is greater emphasis on kicking techniques. However, breaking techniques traditionally play an important role, as does full contact sparring in both training and competition. It is evident that, beyond the need for strength endurance, explosive elastic strength is of paramount importance.

Thai boxing

Thai boxing is closely related to boxing and to the full contact martial arts, so all the necessary safety precautions need to be taken. It also has a religious background, Buddhist philosophy being a very important part of the art for high grades.

Like boxing, emphasis is on sparring, although great use is made of punch bags and pads, shin and foot guards, and gloves. Shadow boxing is included in training, since this is less likely to be hazardous to most students. There is a trend towards development of strength endurance, but for competitions, gradings and lesson periods of sparring elastic strength, and the powerful techniques which it enhances, is critical.

General considerations

It should have become evident that although the various martial arts have differing points of emphasis, they all, in fact, have similar requirements. General strength endurance is essential, if only to enable students to repeat techniques for the length of a lesson. Plyometric strength is of importance with those styles that require explosive action; however, the development of maximum strength seems to be of secondary importance.

Lessons last between one and two hours and are usually divided into periods: warm-up, drills, partner work or sparring, and kata or form work. In general, because of the length of time involved, there is constant activity at a low level of intensity which will develop a basic degree of strength endurance. However, it is the periods of intense work which present the difficulty, since students can manage only short bursts of maximum strength generation without long recovery periods. Training for competition and grading, in which bouts of intense work may continue for two or three minutes at a time, must take into consideration fatigue and recovery.

In summary, endurance and plyometric strength seem to be the key aspects of performance to be developed. Students do not need expensive equipment for this. Their own body weight and the coach's imagination should be sufficient.

In some martial arts 'strengthening' specific parts of the body seems to be a euphemism for enabling a student to withstand pain. Any training which is geared towards reducing a student's sensitivity to pain should not be part of a strength training programme. The toleration of pain is associated with the desensitisation of tissue as a result of damaged nerve receptors, and will increase will-power, and the possibility of injury, rather than develop muscle tissue.

WEIGHT TRAINING FOR THE MARTIAL ARTS

When strength training is mentioned, students and coaches invariably think of using weights. However, for most martial arts clubs weight training equipment is not readily available or, if it is, the range of specialist equipment is limited. Furthermore, martial arts coaches have great expertise in their specific activities, but very few have an adequate background in the technical aspects of lifting weights.

Neither of these shortcomings should deter the conscientious coach. With care, common sense and careful selection of exercises, there should be little risk of injury to student, and to coach! Moreover, although very sophisticated equipment is useful, with a little planning it is not essential. If the coach is still not satisfied with his own ability or equipment after investigating preliminary avenues, there are now many sports centres where specialist facilities and expert advice are easily accessible.

It is not possible within the scope of this book to cover all exercises and the fine elements of specific weight lifting technique. It is my intention to identify examples of the more common activities. The coach must then choose those which are relevant to his martial art or style, since he is the only person with a deep understanding of the requirements.

Arms and upper body

Bench press (1)

The student lies on a bench. The bar is held with arms at least shoulder-width apart. The exercise starts with the bar on the chest. It is then pressed out until the arms are fully extended. (As a safety precaution it is a good idea to use 'spotters' for all exercises. Spotters are training partners who assist by positioning the bar at the start of an exercise and lifting it away at the end. They are also on hand to take the bar if a lift is not completed or if a potentially dangerous situation suddenly arises. Normally two spotters are sufficient, one at either side of the bar.)

Bench press (2)

The same exercise can be performed with two dumb-bells, one in each hand. The starting position is almost the same as for the bench press (1), with the dumb-bells held level with the chest at the start of the exercise. The weights are pressed out simultaneously to full arm extension.

Starting position for bench press (1)

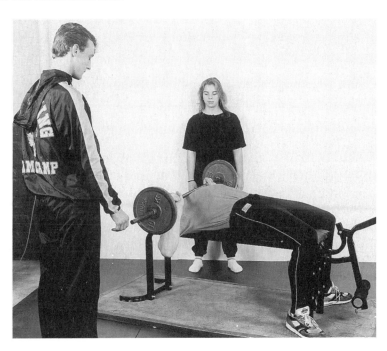

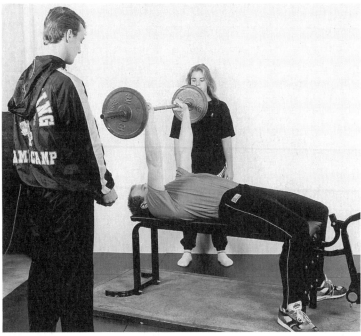

Full extension of the arms in bench press (1). A spotter stands at either side of the student in case he needs assistance

A variation on this exercise is to press out the weights alternately. The lower photograph opposite shows the right arm extended while the left stays in its starting position. As the right arm is lowered, the left is extended. This activity is similar to the action required in some punching techniques. The weights can be rotated as they are pushed away from the chest.

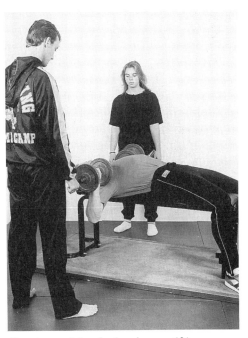

Starting position for bench press (2)

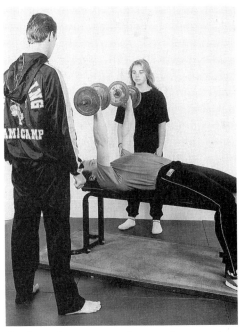

Both weights are pressed out at the same time

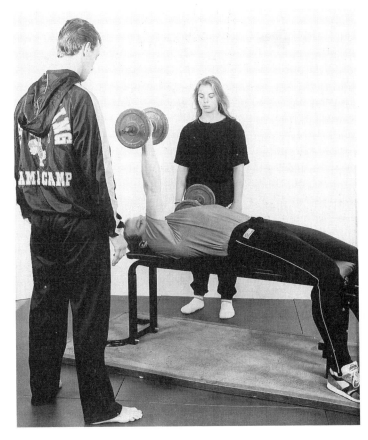

Full extension of the right arm during a variation of bench press (2)

Flying

Lying on a bench with a dumb-bell in each hand, the student takes the weights out to the side of the body, keeping the elbows slightly bent. The arms are then brought together above the chest.

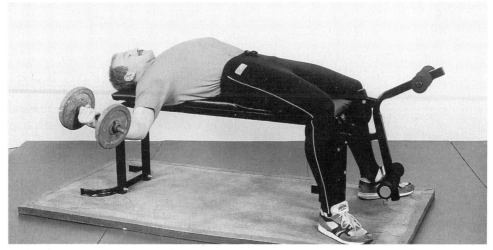

Starting position for the 'flying' exercise

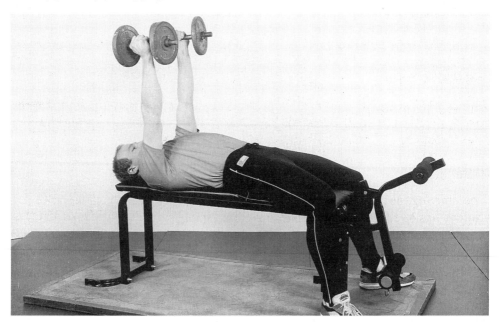

The arms are brought together and straightened above the chest

Military press

Standing with feet shoulder-width apart, the bar is held on the chest. It is then pressed out to full arm extension.

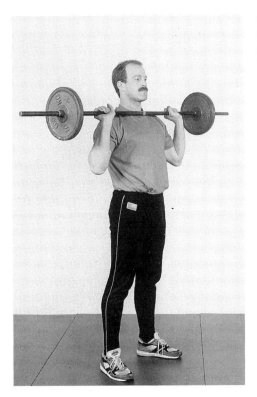 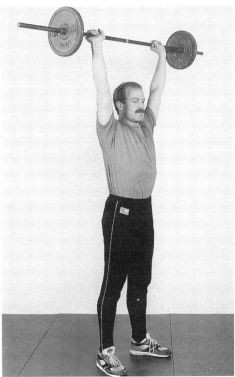

Starting position for the military press   *Full extension of the arms in the military press*

Behind neck press

This is a variation on the military press. The starting position is with the bar resting behind the neck, across the shoulders. Keeping the bar away from and behind the neck, the arms are extended fully.

Neider press

The starting position is very similar to that of the military press, but the student has one foot forward. The bar is not pressed up above the head, but is moved forwards at an angle of about 45 degrees. As a variation, the exercise can be performed with two dumb-bells pressed out simultaneously. A further variant is to press out the dumb-bells alternately.

One modification which the coach might consider is to 'punch' the weights out. The photograph on page 53 (top right) shows a reverse punch-type action. The right and left hands punch forwards alternately. The starting position is with the bar held palm upwards. As the arm is extended, the palm rotates downwards. The coach can modify the angle at which the arm is extended according to the action required. A word of caution: as the weight is punched forwards, care should be taken not to lock out the elbow with undue force. This might cause injury to the joint.

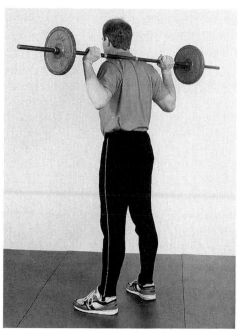

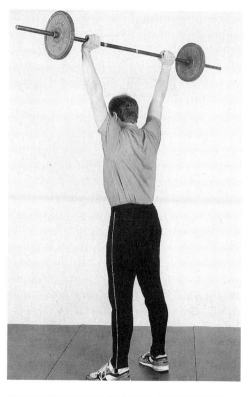

Starting position for the behind neck press

Right *Full extension of the arms in the behind neck press*

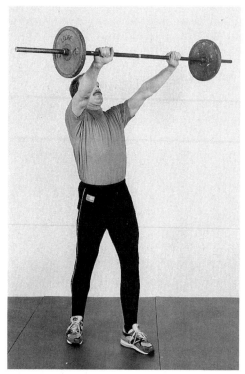

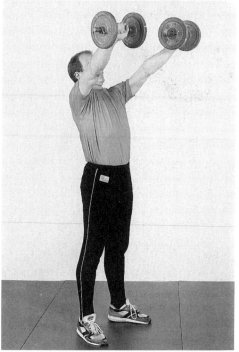

Extended position of the Neider press

Neider press using two dumb-bells simultaneously

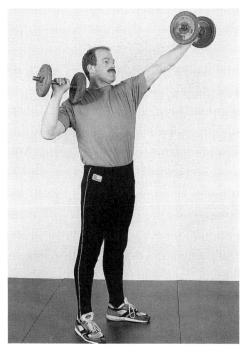

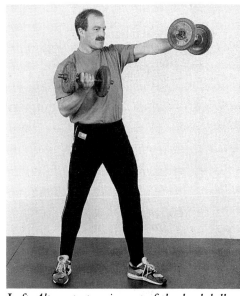

Left *Alternate pressing out of the dumb-bells as a variation of the Neider press*

Above *Reverse punch action using dumb-bells*

French press

A dumb-bell is held with interlocked fingers behind the head and as low as possible. The arms are then extended overhead.

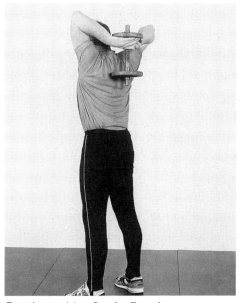

Starting position for the French press

Right *Overhead extension of the arms during the French press*

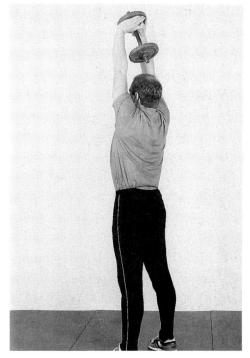

Lateral raises

Two dumb-bells are held at the side of the body. The arms are then lifted outwards until they are at shoulder height.

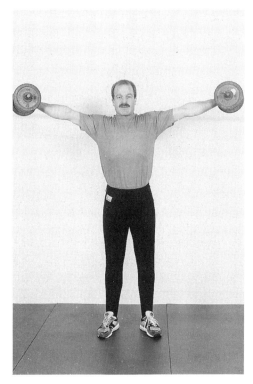

Lateral raise

General exercises

Power cleans

Begin the activity with knees bent, feet underneath the bar, hands shoulder-width apart and, more importantly, keep the back straight. Lift the bar in one movement to the chest. It is essential that the back is kept 'flat' and not 'rounded' throughout the entire lift.

Dead lift

The starting position is the same as for the power clean, but one palm faces forwards and one backwards. The bar is then lifted to waist height, keeping the arms straight.

Straddle dead lift

Stand with one foot in front of, and one behind, the bar, bend down and take hold of the bar. Keeping the arms straight, stand up. Short arms can be a disadvantage in this exercise!

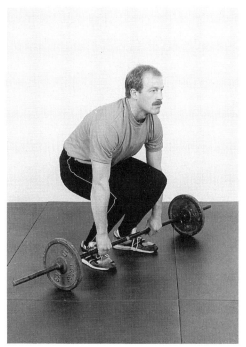

Starting position for power cleans

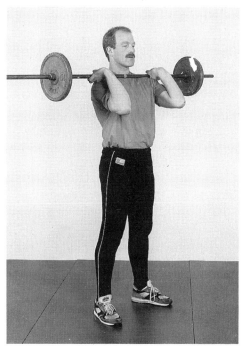

The bar is lifted in one movement to the chest

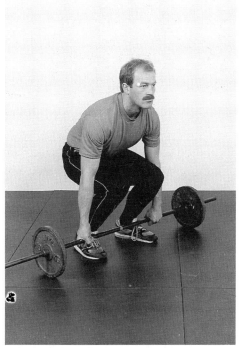

Starting position for the dead lift. Note the placement of the hands on the bar

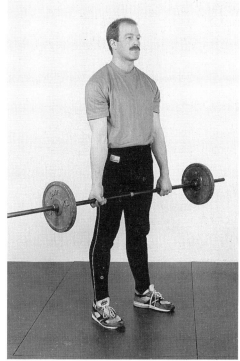

The bar is lifted to waist height

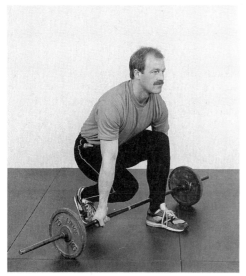

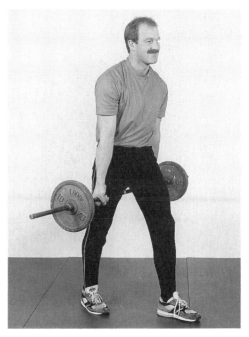

Starting position for the straddle dead lift

Right *The student stands upright and keeps his arms straight*

Hack lift

The starting position is the same as for power cleans, but this time the bar is held behind the ankles. Stand upright, keeping the weight away from the back of the legs.

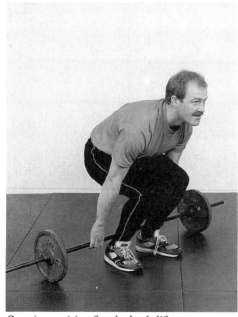

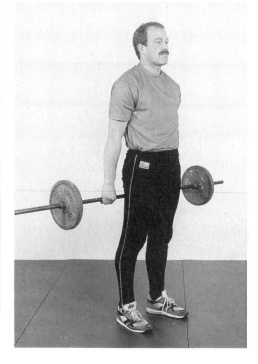

Starting position for the hack lift

Right *Upright position of the hack lift*

Legs

Front squat

Stand with the feet shoulder-width apart, with the bar held across the chest. Bend the knees to approximately 45 degrees. It is not recommended that the knees are bent more than shown in the photograph. Deep squats can put the knees in a mechanically poor position, which could lead to injury.

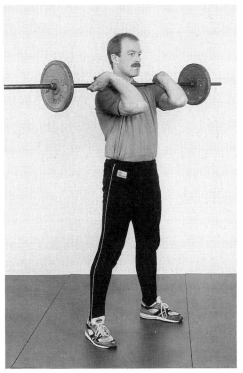

Starting position for front squats

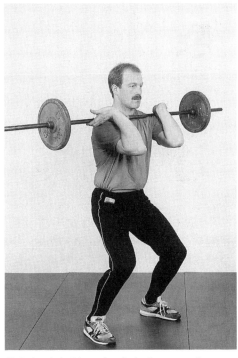

It is inadvisable to bend the knees much more than forty-five degrees

Rear squats

The exercise is very similar to front squats, but the bar is held across the shoulders, behind the head.

Calf raises

As with rear squats, the bar is held across the shoulders, behind the head. Keeping the legs straight, the heels are lifted high off the floor.

Split squats

The bar is held across the shoulders, behind the head. Starting with the right foot forwards and the left foot back, jump as high as possible. Change the position of the legs before landing with the left foot forwards and the right foot back.

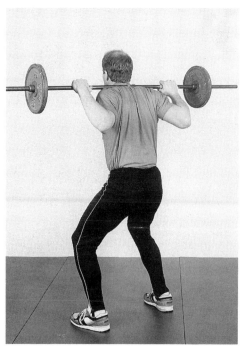

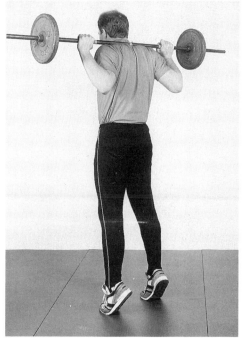

For rear squats, the bar is held behind the head

Calf raise

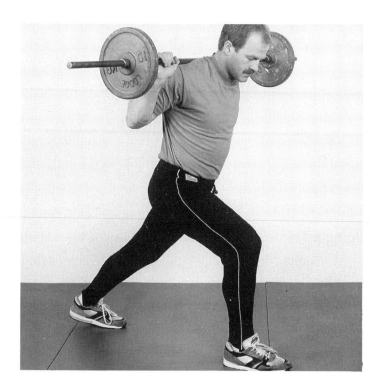

Starting position for jump squats

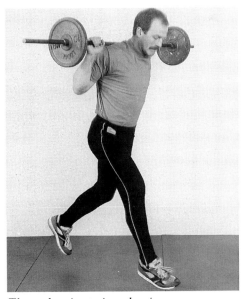
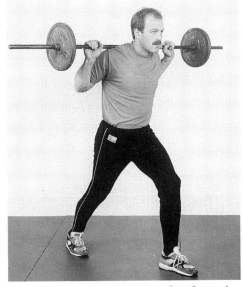

The student jumps into the air . . .   *. . . and lands with the opposite foot forwards*

Jump squats

The bar is held across the shoulders, behind the head, and feet are shoulder-width apart. Bend at the knees slightly (not as much as in the squatting exercises) before jumping off the floor. This activity requires the student immediately on landing to 'rebound' into the next repetition.

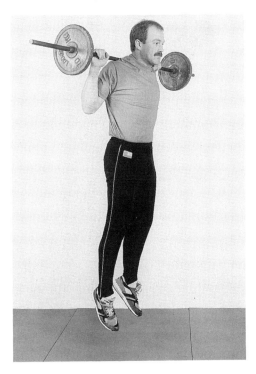

Jump squat

Quad raises

Sit on the edge of the bench, with the feet under the cross-bar. Then lift the feet and straighten the legs.

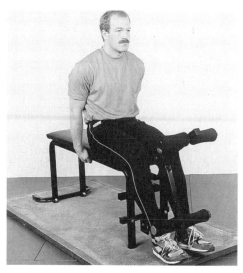

Starting position for quad raises

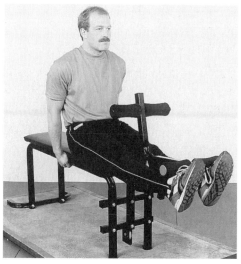

The feet are lifted and the legs are straightened

Hamstring curls

Lying on the bench, hook your heels under the cross-bar. Then bend your knees, lifting the heels high and backwards.

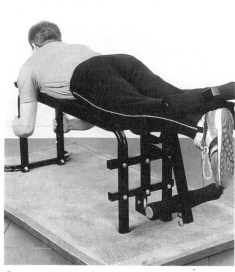

Starting position for hamstring curls

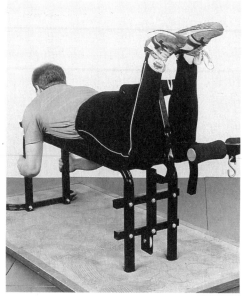

The feet are raised backwards

Abdominal muscles

Sit-ups

Lie on the floor, with a partner holding your feet, keeping your knees slightly bent. Cross your arms over your chest while holding a weight disc. Lift your shoulders approximately 15 cm (6 inches) off the floor.

Bent leg sit-ups

Begin in a similar starting position to sit-ups, but this time keep your knees bent and ensure a partner securely anchors your feet. Again, holding a weight, cross your arms over your chest. Sit up until your elbows just touch your knees.

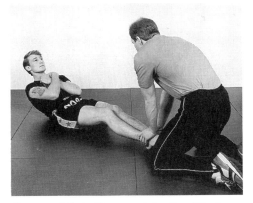

Sit-ups while holding a weight disc. The knees should be kept slightly bent

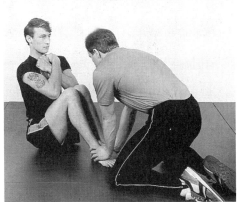

Bent leg sit-ups

Bent leg sit-ups with twist

The starting position is the same as that for bent leg sit-ups, but this time you sit up and twist to allow your right elbow to touch your left knee. On the next sit-up, twist to let the left elbow touch the right knee.

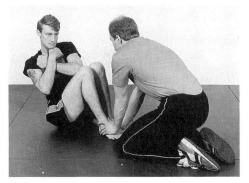

Bent leg sit-up, with the left arm touching the right leg

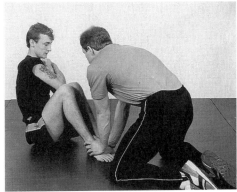

Twisting in the opposite direction

Traditional exercises

Kame

Traditionally, kame or weighted jars were used in highly specific ways to develop strength. There are now, of course, very few modern weight training facilities which boast a selection of differently weighted jars for students to use. However, with a little ingenuity these old exercises can be performed easily in any training hall. The photograph below (left) shows a reverse punch in the horse stance. In each hand is held a weight, in this example a 2.5 kg (5.5 lb) disc. The size of the disc allows the fingers to be wrapped around it to create the desired hand shape, in this instance a claw hand. By varying the size of the weight and the grip a series of hand positions and stances can be developed.

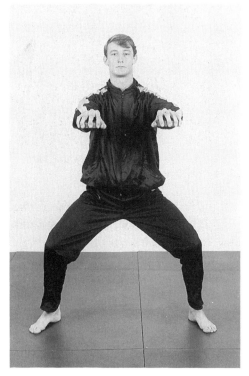
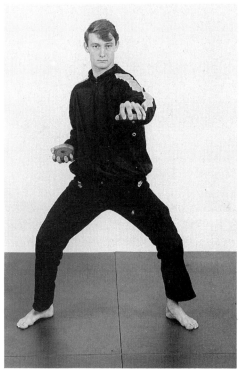

Using hand-held weights and a strong stance to develop strength

Execution of a reverse punch with weights

Shi ishi

Again, shi ishi are not very common, but dumb-bells are. By placing a weight disc at one end of a dumb-bell, with the collars securely fastened, a modern day version of shi ishi can be produced. The main theme behind these traditional exercises was to develop highly specific strength. The photographs opposite show a classic exercise, once again in horse stance. The dumb-bells are held, weight down, at arm's length, and the palms are twisted outwards. The dumb-bells are then turned inwards and upwards.

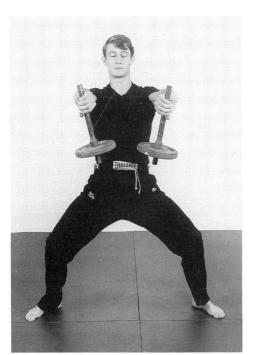 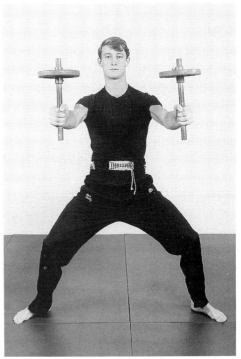

Modern day version of shi ishi. The dumb-bells are held with the weights down and the palms of the hands twisted outwards

Keeping the horse stance, the dumb-bells are moved inwards and upwards

Most coaches and students of the martial arts are great readers of the historical development of their particular style. Many books have descriptions of traditional exercises, together with copies of paintings and drawings depicting training exercises. It should be relatively straightforward to adapt some of the more enlightened practices to modern equipment. For example, the tan or weighted bar is very similar to the barbell. A bar 6 ft (1.8 m) in length weighs 10 kg (22 lb); a standard Olympic bar with collars weighs 25 kg (44 lb). By adding or subtracting weights and conscientiously securing the collars, bars appropriate to any strength level or exercise can easily be produced. The limit to the range of exercises in this case depends upon the research skills of student and coach.

WEIGHT TRAINING WITH A PARTNER

It may seem an odd comment to make, but it is quite possible to perform many exercises that usually require sophisticated and expensive equipment by replacing them with a partner! Some of these activities are classic 'weightlifting' exercises and are modified simply by another student's weight or resistance being used instead of weight discs. The only limitation to this type of 'weight training' is the imagination of the coach. In other exercises described a partner is a helpful aid, both as an incentive to training and as a useful immovable object.

Biceps curls

The photographs show the classic biceps curl. However, a partner can help produce exactly the same loading on the muscles. He kneels in front of the student so that they can interlink fingers. Keeping the upper arm fixed, the

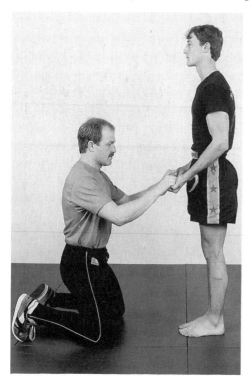

Starting position for biceps curls

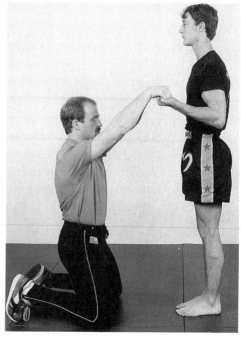

The standing student moves his hands towards his chest, keeping his upper arms in the same position

hands are moved up towards the chest. The advantage of this type of training is that the coach can identify the exact type of load and muscle action to be used, as well as the range of movement.

Lateral raises

The arms are held straight and down by the sides. They are then lifted out to the side until they are level with the shoulders. The partner once again varies the load as required. Compare this exercise with lateral raises on page 54.

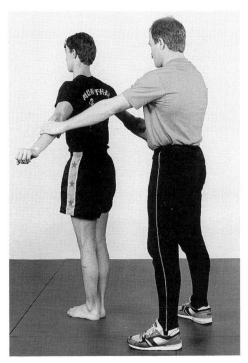

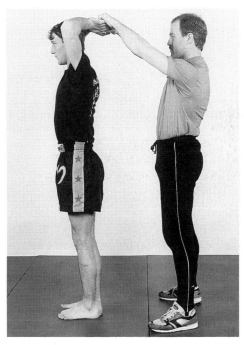

French press with the help of a partner. Compare this illustration with the photographs at the bottom of page 53

Lateral raise. Compare this illustration with the photograph on page 54

French press

The partner stands behind the student, providing the resistance. Compare this with the French press on page 53.

Press-ups

In a normal press-up position, the student places his feet on the back of his partner. He performs the exercise to straighten the arms fully. Obviously more weight is being placed upon the arms than in the normal press-up, which makes this variation more difficult. It should be clear that the muscle action is almost identical to that for the bench press (see page 65), but in this example the student is facing down, not up!

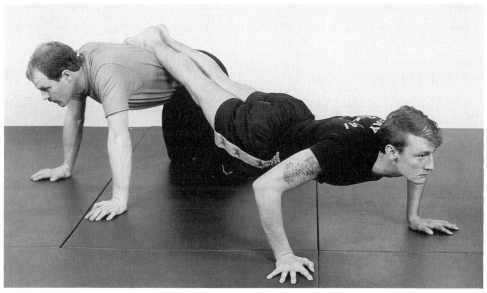

Press-ups, with the student's feet supported by his partner's back

Leg raises

The student lies on his back with his feet towards a partner. Keeping both legs straight, he raises them to touch his hands. The partner can vary the effort needed by raising or lowering his hands. He can also resist the legs being raised by gently pushing down on them.

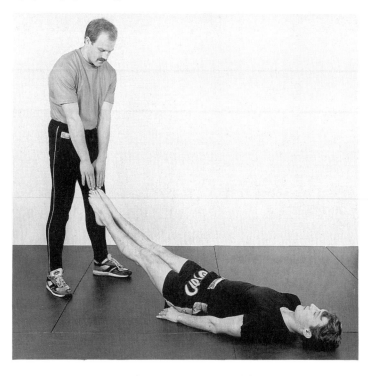

Leg raises

Shoulder raises

Start by lying on your front, with your hands behind your head and your feet securely anchored by a partner. Lift your chest as far away from the floor as possible.

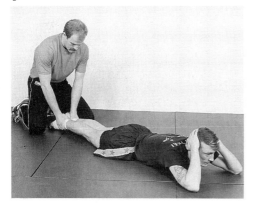

Shoulder raises

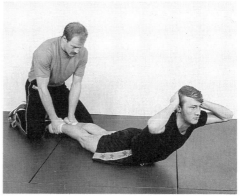

The student performing the exercise must raise his chest from the floor at the same time keeping his hands behind his head

Leg raises

These are a variation on shoulder raises. Lying on your front, with your hands behind your neck, a partner should firmly press your chest to the floor. Keeping your legs straight, lift them high off the floor.

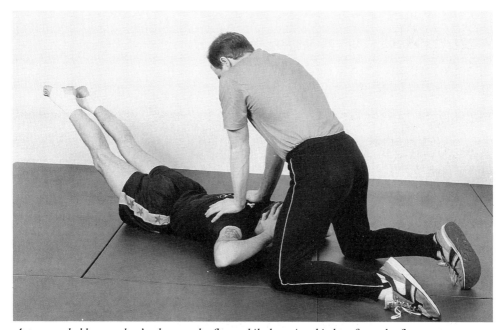

A partner holds a student's chest to the floor while he raises his legs from the floor

Double leg press

Lie on your back, with your hands behind your neck, feet raised and knees bent. A partner should lean forwards so that his chest rests upon your feet. Your legs should then be straightened with force.

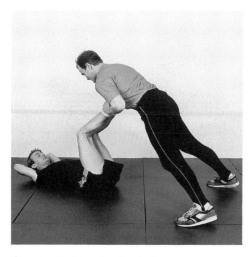

Starting position for double leg press

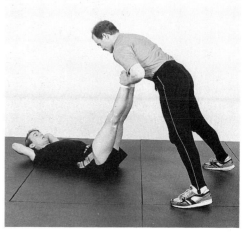

The student lying on the floor straightens his legs against his partner who partly resists the movement

Single leg press

The starting position is the same as that for the double leg press, but in this exercise only one leg is used at a time. The first photograph shows the beginning of the action with the left leg. The leg is then straightened (see second photograph). The exercise is repeated using the right leg.

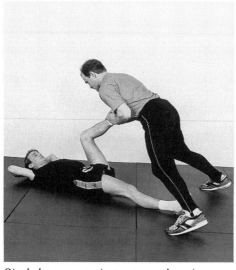

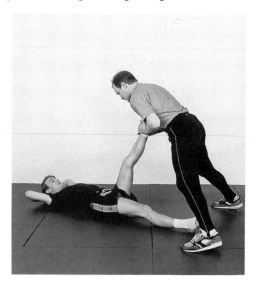

Single leg press against a partner's resistance

Hamstring curls

Lie on your front, with your legs extended. Your partner should kneel down and take hold of your ankles. By bending your knees, your heels will be lifted as high and far back towards your thighs as possible.

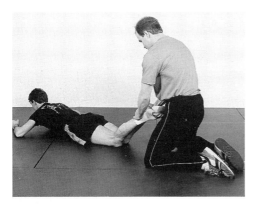

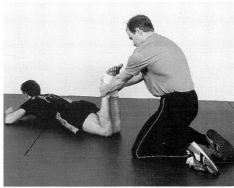

Hamstring curl. The knees are bent until . . .   *. . . the heels are as near the thighs as possible*

Squats

Stand back to back with a partner, with your elbows interlinked. Carefully squat down until your thighs are parallel to the floor.

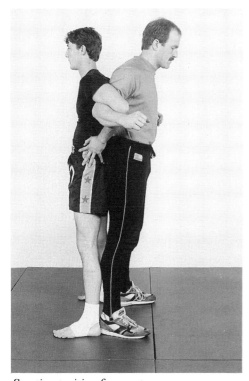

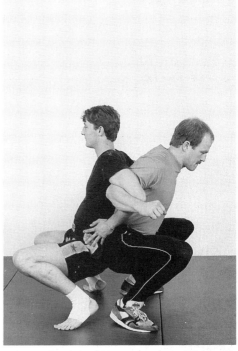

The students should try to keep their backs as straight as possible

Starting position for squats

Leg push

Sit facing a partner, bend your knees and lift your feet off the floor so that the soles of your feet are touching. Your hands should be placed behind your body for support. You should try to straighten your legs by forcing your partner to bend his.

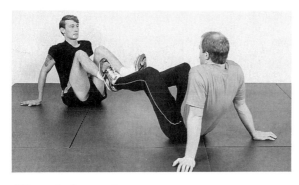

Starting position for leg push

Alternate leg push

The starting position is the same as that for the leg push. With this exercise the students take it in turns to straighten their legs.

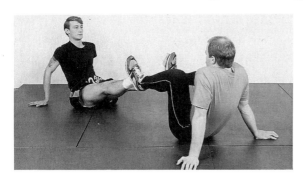

One student straightens his legs while the other bends his legs

Single alternate leg push

The starting position is the same as that for the alternate leg push. The aim of this exercise is to extend one leg at a time.

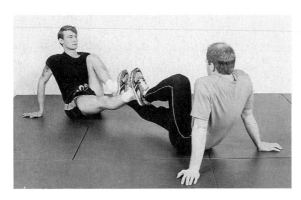

Alternate leg push

BODY WEIGHT

Much strength training for the martial arts uses the most basic item of equipment, the student's own body! The logic behind this is quite simple. During the course of a normal lesson it would be impractical constantly to bring out and put away equipment; bodies are far more convenient and readily available. It therefore falls to the coach to devise appropriate exercises, and therein lies the root of many problems. A busy coach does not have the time to prepare individual programmes for each student, the consequence of which is all students practising the same exercises at each lesson. Boredom can soon ensue.

This section looks at some of the more commonly used exercises and suggests a few variations to help maintain the students' interest.

Press-ups

Press-ups are perhaps the most popular strength training exercise. With a little ingenuity the effect on muscle groups, as well as on the students' enthusiasm, can be changed.

Narrow press-ups (1)

The starting position is with the arms held straight and the index fingers and thumbs touching. Bend your arms so that your nose touches the floor in the triangle created by your thumbs and index fingers.

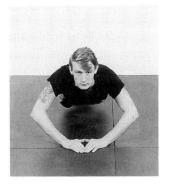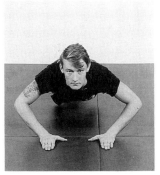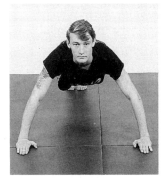

Starting position for narrow press-ups. The hands are gradually moved further and further apart

Narrow press-ups (2)

Move each hand one 'hand's width' away. You can continue to do this until you reach the hand position for the 'standard' press-up. This hand spacing can now be the starting position for:

Wide press-ups (1)

Move each hand a further 'hand's width' away. Again, this procedure can be followed until the hands are as far away from each other as can be managed.

Each of these press-up examples can be selected by the coach as a specific exercise, or the series can be performed in sequence, working from the narrow to the wide version in a mini-circuit. A further variation of the press-up is to move the hands forwards.

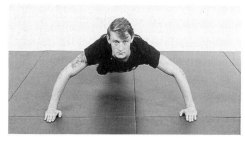

Starting position for wide press-ups

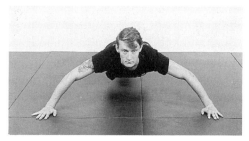

The hands are moved further and further apart

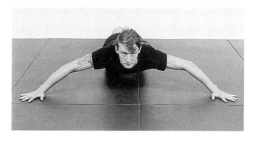

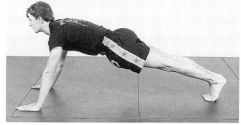

Normal starting position for the standard press-up

Extended press-ups (1)

The starting position is achieved by moving the hands one 'hand's length' forwards.

For extended press-ups the hands can be moved further and further forwards

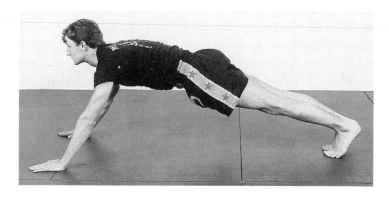

Extended press-ups (2)

Move the hands a further 'hand's length' forwards. Continue moving the hands as far forwards as possible.

As with the narrow to wide press-ups, each of these exercises can be selected individually or can be performed sequentially as a mini-circuit. The same is true of the following exercises.

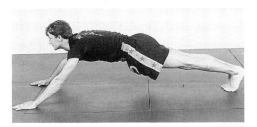 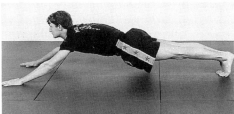

Reverse press-ups (1)

The starting position is the same as that for the standard press-up, but the hands are positioned in such a way that the fingers point towards the student's feet.

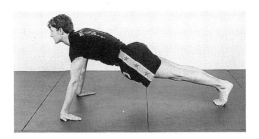

Starting position for reverse press-ups

Reverse press-ups (2)

Move your hands one 'hand's length' towards your feet. Continue in the same fashion, each time moving your hands towards your feet.

If the coach takes the opportunity to try some of the variations on press-ups which have been described, he will notice that each one affects a different group of muscles. With a little modification an exercise as simple as a press-up

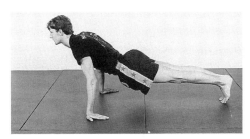 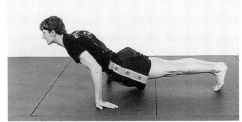

The hands are gradually moved back

can work in a very specific way most, if not every muscle group in the arms, chest and shoulders. The variations ought to be selected for their effect by the coach, although I would tend to favour the circuit idea which covers each variation sequentially. In this way all muscle groups are worked, thereby giving a balanced development of strength.

Further variations on press-ups are as follows:

Snappers

Most students at some time will have practised the hand clap press-up in which the upper body is pushed away from the floor explosively to give the hands time to be brought together before resuming their normal position on the floor. For snappers hands and feet start shoulder-width apart. On the push phase they leave the floor. The hands are clapped and the heels are brought together before landing in the original position.

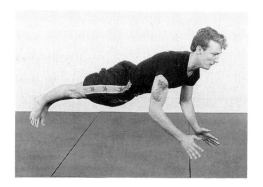

For snappers the hands and feet are brought together in mid-air

Hand walk (1)

The starting position is the same as for the standard press-up, but the feet are kept together. Pivoting on the balls of his feet, the student then walks on his hands in an anti-clockwise direction until he arrives at the starting position. Movement can be in a clockwise direction as well.

Students can imagine their feet as the fixed point in a pair of compasses and their hands as the pencil drawing out the circle. A variation on this exercise is the hand walk.

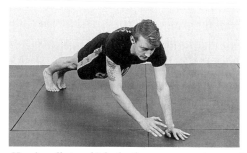 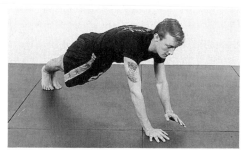

Hand walk in which the feet act as a pivot and the hands describe a circle

Hand walk (2)

In this exercise the hands act as the pivot and the feet draw out a large circle in an anti-clockwise, or clockwise, direction.

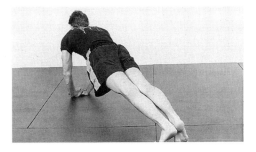
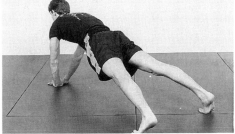

Hand walk in which the hands act as the pivot and the feet describe a circle

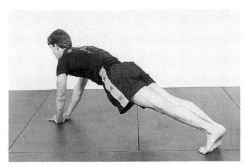

Seal walk

This activity really is a combination of all of the exercises described so far. In the starting position the weight of the legs is taken on the toes. Keeping their legs straight and dragging them behind, the students walk forwards on their hands.

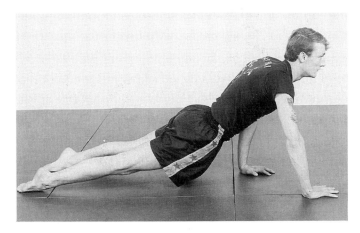

The seal walk

Body curls

Lie on your back, with your knees slightly bent and your hands on your thighs. Raise your upper body until your fingers just touch your knees.

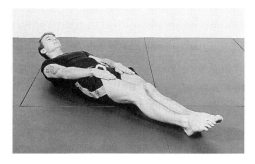

Starting position for body curls

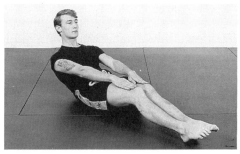

Keeping the knees slightly bent, the body is raised so that the fingers touch the knees

Bent leg sit-ups

Lie on your back, with your hands at the sides of your head, your knees bent and your feet shoulder-width apart. Raise your upper body until your elbows just touch your knees.

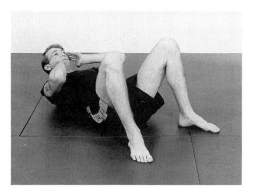

Starting position for bent leg sit-ups

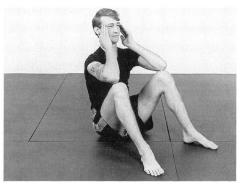

The upper body is raised until the elbows touch the knees

Bent leg sit-ups with twist

The starting position is the same as for bent leg sit-ups. As the upper body is raised, the left elbow is brought across to touch the right knee. The exercise is repeated, twisting the right elbow across to the left knee.

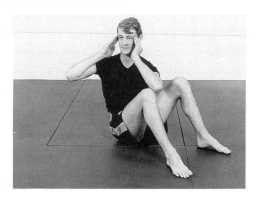

Bent leg sit-up with twist

Trunk twisters

Sit with your knees bent. Lift your right knee; at the same time lift and turn your upper body to allow your left elbow to touch it. The exercise is repeated by turning the right elbow across to touch the left knee.

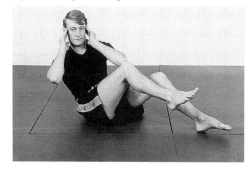

Trunk twister

'V'-sits

Lie on your back, with your arms and legs fully extended. Simultaneously throw your arms forwards and lift your legs so that your hands touch your feet.

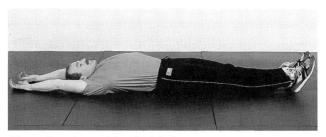
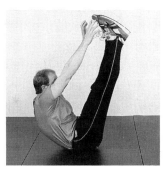

Above *Starting position for 'v'-sits*
Right *The student tries to bring arms and legs together*

Double leg circling

Lie on your back, with your hands down by your sides for support. Keeping your legs straight, lift them off the floor and move them in an anti-clockwise direction. The less the feet are raised, the greater the effect.

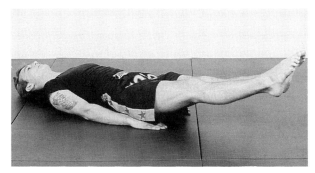

Double leg circling

Single leg circling

The starting position is the same as for double leg circling, but the legs are wide apart. From this position the feet are circled in an anti-clockwise direction. The exercise is repeated, circling the feet in a clockwise direction.

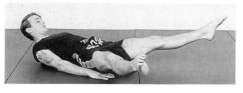

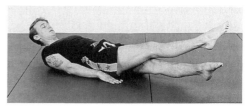

The feet are circled in both directions during single leg circling

Crossing of the legs during scissors

Scissors

The starting position is the same as for single leg circling. The legs are brought together, right over left, before being moved out wide again. The exercise is repeated, taking the left leg over the right leg.

Jump squats

Stand with the feet shoulder-width apart. Jump as high as possible while bringing the knees to the chest.

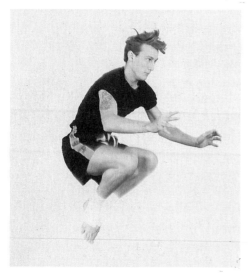

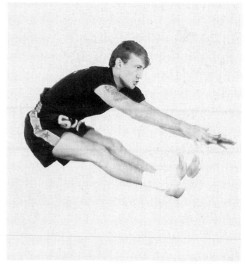

Jump squat, bringing the knees to the chest

Piked jump, with the legs straight out in front

Piked jumps

Stand with the feet shoulder-width apart. Jump as high as possible, but this time lift the legs straight out in front while at the same time trying to touch the toes with the fingers.

Split squats

Kneel down, left foot forward and right foot back, with the hands on the floor for support. Jump as high as possible and while in the air change the position of the feet. Land with the right foot forward and the left foot back. It is important that the arms should be used to help cushion the landing. The exercise is repeated, changing the position of the feet each time.

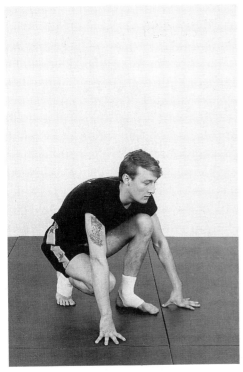 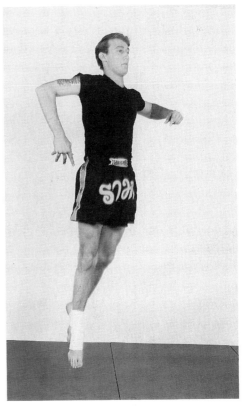

Left *Starting position for split squats*
Right *The student jumps into the air and . . .*

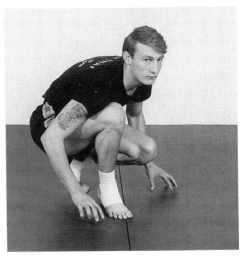

. . . lands in the opposite stance

Treadmill

In an almost press-up position, place the left foot between the hands so that the knee is bent to a right angle. Drive the left leg straight backwards, at the same time bringing the right foot forwards to land between the hands; the knee is bent at right angles. The exercise is repeated, changing the position of the feet each time.

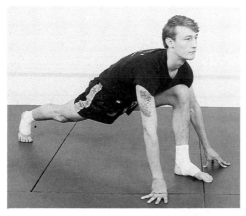

Treadmill starting with the left leg forward

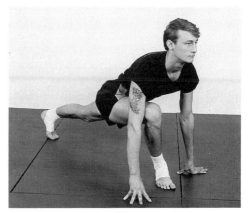

The left leg is pushed back and the right leg is brought forward

Squat thrusts

Squat on the floor, with the hands at the side for support. The legs are driven straight back to full extension, before being drawn forwards again to land between the hands.

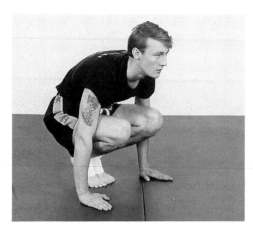

Starting position for squat thrusts

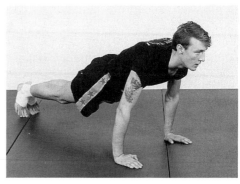

The legs are driven straight back

IMPROVISATION AND VARIATIONS

As we have seen, sophisticated equipment, although extremely helpful, is not essential: a partner's resistance and a student's own body weight can be used to great effect. Similarly, readily available items of equipment, and furniture, can with a little imagination provide an alternative programme of strength development. A few ideas to set coaches thinking are described in the following examples.

Chair press

The starting position and whole movement are the same as those for a standard press-up, but with each hand on a chair. The effort required can be made greater by placing the feet on a chair, too.

Chair dips

Sit with your back to a chair, hands firmly holding either side of the seat. Lift your body off the floor by straightening your arms. The effect of the exercise can be increased by raising the feet onto either another chair or the back of a partner. As a point of safety it is recommended that a partner holds the back of the chair to prevent it from tipping forwards.

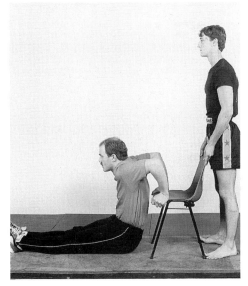

Starting position for chair dips

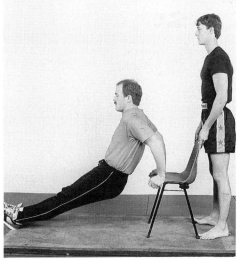

The arms are straightened to lift the body off the floor

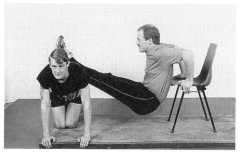

Increasing the effect of chair dips by placing the feet on a partner's back

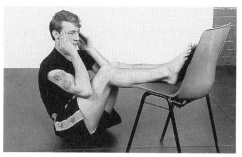

Chair sit-up

Chair sit-ups

Lie on the floor, with your legs on the seat of a chair and knees bent. With your hands held at the side of your head, sit up until your elbows touch your knees.

Step-ups

Stand facing a chair. Lift your left leg to place your foot on the seat of the chair. Moving your weight forwards, stand on the chair by bringing your right foot up to join the left. Step down, left foot first, followed by the right. The exercise is repeated, leading both the step up and down with the right leg. Again, for safety purposes, it is best if a partner holds the back of the chair.

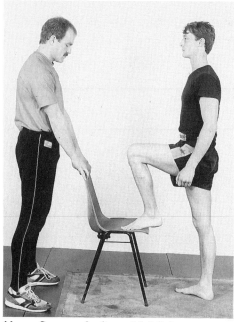

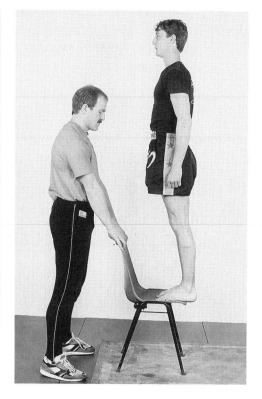

Above Step-up, leading with left leg
Right For safety purposes it is best if a partner holds the chair while the exercise is being performed

Inclined sit-ups

Lying on the bench, hook your feet under the cross bar. Holding your hands at the side of your head, sit up until your elbows touch your knees.

Inclined sit-ups with twist

The starting position is the same as for inclined sit-ups. As the body moves forwards, the left elbow is twisted across to touch the right knee. The exercise is repeated, twisting the right elbow across to the left knee.

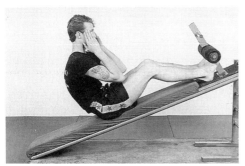

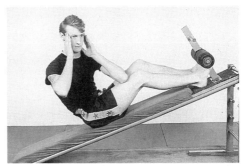

Inclined sit-up, keeping the knees slightly bent to avoid injury to the back

Inclined sit-up with twist

Weighted inclined sit-ups

The starting position and action are exactly the same as for the inclined sit-up. This time the student holds a weight disc, with arms crossed on the chest. A medicine ball can be used instead of a weight disc.

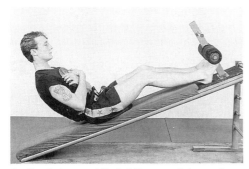

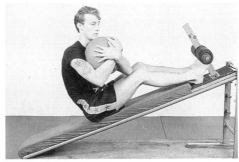

Inclined sit-up while holding a weight against the chest

Inclined sit-up while holding a medicine ball

Inclined leg raises

Lie on your back holding the cross bar for support. A partner should stand facing you, with arms held downwards. Lift your feet to touch the partner's hands. The exercise can be made more difficult if you hold a medicine ball between your feet.

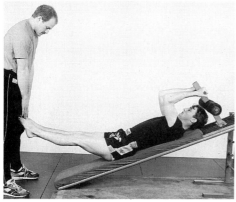

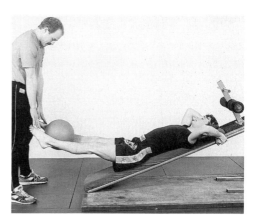

Above, left *Starting position for inclined leg raises*
Above, right *A medicine ball can be held between the feet to make the exercise more difficult*

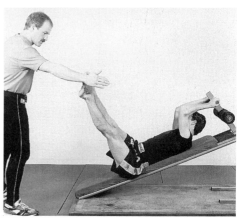

The legs are raised until they touch the partner's outstretched hand

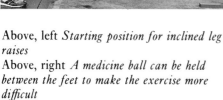

Inclined hip twisters

The starting position is the same as that for inclined leg raises. In this exercise the partner stands to the left of the bench, with his arms outstretched. While keeping his shoulders on the bench, the student twists at the hips to raise both feet to touch his partner's hands. The exercise is repeated, but with the partner standing on the right.

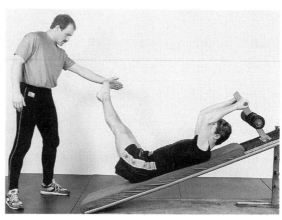

Hip twister to the right

Astride jumps

Stand on a bench with your feet together. Jump down to land with one foot either side of the bench. On landing, immediately 'rebound' to jump back on the bench.

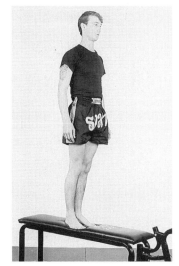

Starting position for astride jumps

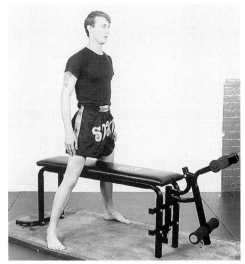

On landing astride the bench, the student immediately jumps back onto it

Squat jumps

Stand on the right side of a bench, firmly holding the top with both hands. Jump high over it to land on the left side. Repeat the exercise immediately on landing by jumping back to the right side.

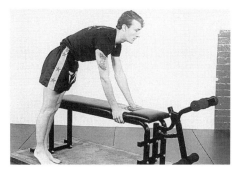

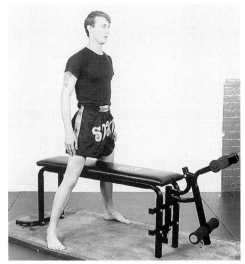

Starting position for squat jumps
Right *The student jumps over the bench . . .*

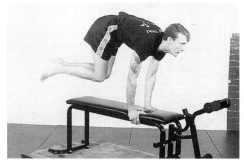

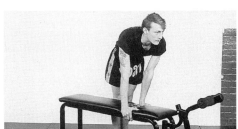

. . . to land on the opposite side

Bunny hops (1)

The student stands at the right side of a line of canes supported by cones or a long bench. Keeping both feet together, jump up and over the canes to land on the left side. On landing, immediately rebound and jump back to the right side. As you jump from side to side, also move along the length of the canes or bench.

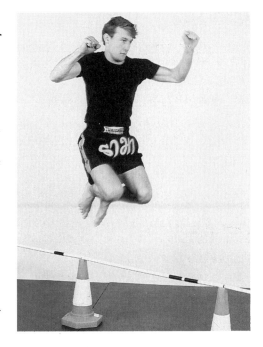

Jumping over a cane, keeping both feet together; the exercise can be varied by jumping from one leg to another

Bunny hops (2)

The starting position and the action are the same as those for bunny hops (1). However, this time hop over the canes or bench on the right leg and then repeat the exercise using the left leg.

Bunny hops (3)

With this variation the cones are set out like hurdles. The student jumps with both feet together over the sequence of canes. Students can also hop on their right leg over the canes and then repeat the exercise using their left leg.

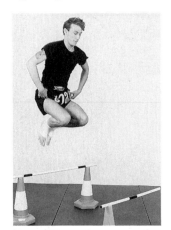
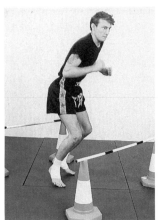
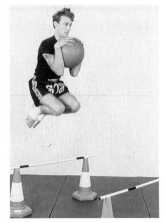

Above *The student jumps high over each hurdle*
Right *Jumping with a medicine ball makes the exercise more difficult to execute*

Bunny hops (4)

As a further variation, the activity can be made more difficult and effective if the student holds a medicine ball or a weight.

Medicine ball kick (1)

Lie on your back, with your legs raised, knees slightly bent, and your feet together. A partner should throw a medicine ball so that it lands on the soles of your feet. As the ball just touches them, kick it back to your partner.

Medicine ball kick (2)

The starting position and the action are similar to those of Medicine ball kick (1). This time only the left leg is used. The exercise is repeated using the right leg.

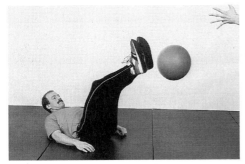

Medicine ball kick with two feet

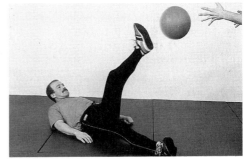

Medicine ball kick with one foot

Hamstring curls

Lie on the floor on your front. A partner should stand over your back so that he can roll a medicine ball down the back of your legs. As it touches your ankles, flick it back to your partner.

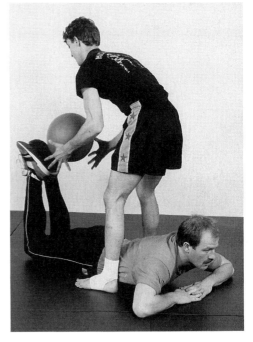

Hamstring curl

Chest pass (1)

Face a partner, holding a medicine ball in both hands on your chest with your elbows out to your side. Push the ball to your partner, giving a final flick with the fingers. Your partner should throw it back in a similar fashion.

Chest pass (2)

Facing a partner, hold a medicine ball in your left hand and use the right for support. Push the ball towards your partner, who should return it in a similar fashion. Repeat the exercise using the right hand.

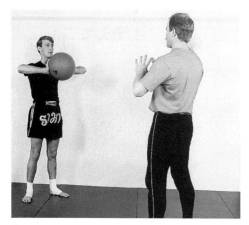

Starting position for the chest pass

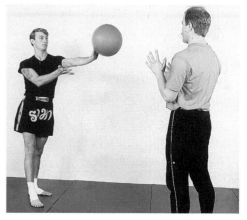

To vary the chest pass, throw with just one hand and support the throwing arm with the other arm

Knee drive

A partner carefully throws a medicine ball so that the student can 'knee' it upwards, using the right leg. As an alternative action, the ball can be driven forwards. The exercise can be repeated using the left leg.

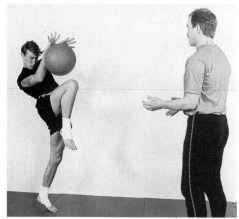

The student propels the medicine ball upwards using his right knee

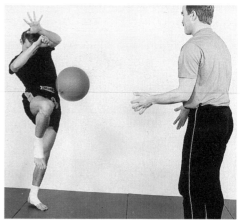

In this exercise the ball is sent forwards by the right knee

Medicine ball kick

A partner throws a medicine ball so that the student can kick it back using the right leg. The exercise is repeated using the left leg. The partner can vary the direction and height of the throw to develop different kicks.

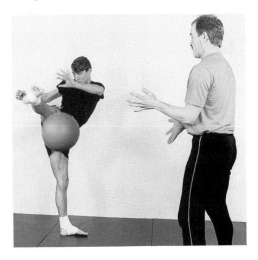

Various kicks can be used to return the ball to a partner

Kicks

By carefully attaching a rope around your foot and having a partner standing behind to offer a variable resistance, a series of kicks can be practised with the right or left leg.

Punches

In a similar fashion to the kicking activities, punches can be developed using the right or left hand.

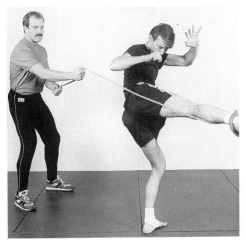

Practising kicks with the aid of a rope and a partner

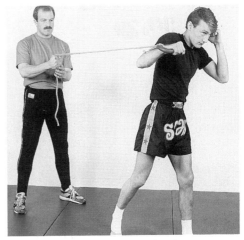

Punches can also be practised with a partner and a piece of rope

SAFE TRAINING

With strength training in particular extra precautions have to be taken to ensure the safety of the students.

- The training area must be kept clear of items of equipment at all times. Each student should have adequate space in which to train; overcrowding must not be allowed to develop.
- All equipment must be regularly maintained and inspected.
- When loose weights are used, all weight discs must be held secure by collars.
- Where appropriate, training partners should be available to lift the weight on or off or to stand by during the exercise.
- Good lifting technique should be practised at all times.
- A thorough warm-up should precede any form of strength training.
- Young students should develop general strength. There is no reason why they should use loads heavier than their own body weight.
- The back must be kept straight in all lifting activities.
- Any activity must be stopped if a student feels pain in the area being worked.
- Injuries to the knees can occur if they are bent too much. A very low position brought about by squatting or bending the knees as much as possible is not advisable, especially when a load is used.
- Make sure that there is sufficient rest between exercises to allow full recovery. After intensive strength training, tissues lose their elasticity. It is therefore not advisable to work to the same level again in any training session.

GOOD PRACTICE

Any martial art or demanding physical activity requires a series of safety measures to ensure that all those students involved can train in the best possible conditions.

Coach education programme

The Martial Arts Commission (MAC) of Great Britain has devised a comprehensive coach education programme which is run in conjunction with the major martial arts governing bodies. Potential students or parents should check the qualifications of an instructor to provide efficient, effective and safe teaching. Any coach who possesses a MAC coaching qualification demonstrates competence as an instructor.

Legal implications

One has only to read the 'court' columns in the newspapers to appreciate that there is recourse to the law to obtain compensation for a wide range of injuries. It is vital that in a potentially dangerous activity, such as the martial arts, each individual is fully insured. Again, I would advise a potential student to contact the MAC or the appropriate governing body for details. Insurance falls into four broad areas.

Student-to-student insurance

This covers students for personal injury that might occur when training with other students under the watchful eye of the instructor.

Dental insurance

Most martial arts put students at risk from damage to teeth. This type of injury is not included in the student-to-student policy and requires additional cover.

Club insurance

Martial arts clubs usually use either a local authority facility or their own building. It is essential that adequate insurance is taken out to cover the loss of personal effects and injury caused by building defects.

Professional indemnity

Any person who coaches must have insurance cover. There is no difference in law between a 'professional' and an 'amateur' coach: both must be covered. A student who instructs other students or groups must also possess professional indemnity. Student-to-student cover is not applicable when a student teaches.

Assessment of students

Before students join a club or organisation, it is prudent for the coach to interview them. An informal meeting allows the instructor to identify students' reasons for wanting to train. It also provides an opportunity for health problems to be discussed.

Recommendations

There are specific criteria which the facilities used for training must meet. The MAC has identified the following guidelines.

- The minimum recommended mat size is $5.5 \, \text{m} \times 5.5 \, \text{m}$ (6 yd $\times$ 6 yd).
- For individual practice, each student requires $3 \, \text{m}^2$ (3yd^2).
- Each student should perform katas in $4 \, \text{m}^2$ ($4\frac{3}{8} \, \text{yd}^2$).
- Sparring, randori or free practice require $11 \, \text{m}^2$ ($12 \, \text{yd}^2$).
- There should be a minimum of 3 m (3 yd) of clear space between the floor and the ceiling. More is advisable when weapons are used.
- The floor should be free from damaged or protruding floor boards or nails. At all times it must be clean and clear of items of clothing or equipment. Any activities which require the use of mats must have: (a) the officially recognised mats for that style, and (b) no damage to or gaps between the mats.
- Any pillars, radiators or other fixtures close to the training area must be sufficiently padded. Mirrors, like any type of glass, should be at least 2 m (2 yd) away from the activity and should be protected.

Maintenance of equipment

Items of equipment, such as kick or punch pads and weapons, must be looked after properly and must be checked prior to each session.

Personal care

Students entering the training area should not wear jewellery, or have sharp nails or torn or damaged clothing which might cause injury. In addition, as a point of safety, all cuts should be covered and personal hygiene should be of the highest standard.

As part of its brief, the MAC provides advice and information on any or all of the above professional, organisational, administrative and legal requirements. I would recommend any student or parent to contact the MAC if they have queries concerning effective and safe instruction.

The physical dimension

Once in the lesson, there are further practices to be followed to ensure the safe training of all students.

Warm-up

It is essential that there is a warm-up period to prepare the students for the intense work which is to follow. The warm-up must be appropriate to the age, sex and fitness level of each individual; for a 'mixed' group this can prove difficult unless it is well designed.

Juniors

Junior martial artists, generally those under 16 years of age, need special consideration when their training is being devised, because their vital organs, such as the heart, lungs and liver, and their muscles and bones are still growing. The difficulty is to identify a work load which will allow students to adapt to different types of training without causing structural damage.

Overloading

The greatest potential for injury in the young student is linked to the skeletal system, joints, ligaments, tendons and associated muscle. Bones are not fully mature until the early twenties; any overloading of joints can bring about structural damage which falls into the following areas.

Structural damage to the bones that make up the joint, because they are 'soft' and cannot cope with either high loads or sustained periods of effort. Particular care must be taken not to overload the spine.

Inflammation or damage to the growth plates at the end of the bones. The main long bones of the body grow from the ends; any damage to these very delicate areas can result in soreness or, in extreme cases, can stop growth altogether.

Ligaments are designed to keep bones at joints in correct alignment. Any attempt to overstretch them can make a joint unstable.

The **muscles** of young students are best suited to long periods of moderately low intensity work. Any attempt to introduce sustained periods of intense activity will rapidly bring about fatigue, which itself could lead to injury.

There has to be a **careful balance** between work and recovery for the young student. Since tissues are still growing, their ability to tolerate work will be less than those in adults. Juniors, therefore, must have periods of low activity interspersed with intense work to allow proper recovery.

With **mobility exercises** any attempt to increase the range of movement at a joint must be accompanied by strengthening activities for the surrounding muscles to help keep the joint stable.

Women do not respond to heavy training in the same way that men do. In general, the training for females has to be increased more gradually than for men, since their bodies adapt to work loads at a slightly slower rate (see Fig. 14). With skill learning, there is little difference between the sexes in the rate at which they improve. It should be remembered that in female students over the age of 45 years there may be a tendency for the skeletal system to degenerate as the result of an inability to tolerate the excesses of training.

Allowances should be made in the training programme for the ageing process. By the age of 25, students will have reached physical maturity (see Fig.

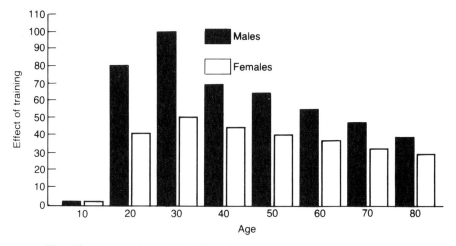

Fig. 13 *A comparison of the effect of training with respect to age and sex*

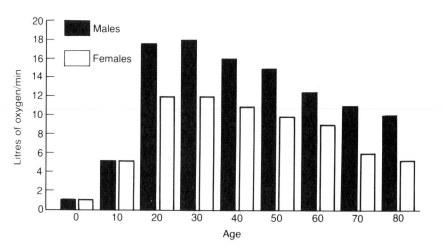

Fig. 14 *A comparison of work rate with respect to age and sex*

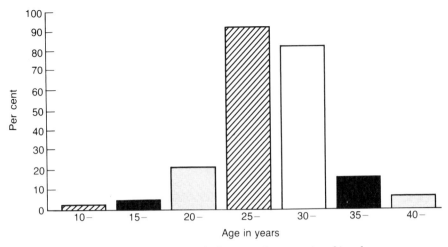

Fig. 15 *The age at which top performance is achieved*

15); thereafter performance will tend to decline. It is important, therefore, that exercises are devised to counter these problems.

Fig. 16 shows the level of improvement that can be expected through training. Although all students can increase their performance, the degree to which they can do so diminishes with age. If this is not realised by the more mature students, frustration can set in.

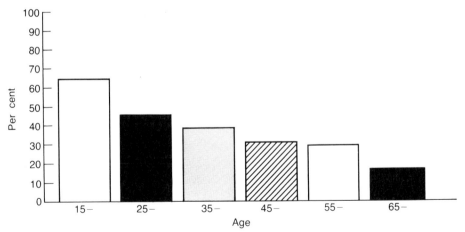

Fig. 16 *The degree of possible improvement with age*

INDEX